The Physics & Poetry of

EASTERN HERBAL MEDICINE

Judyth Shamosh

PH.D., SYSTEMS HERBALIST

For press inquiries, contact the author at http://www.judythshamosh.com/

First Edition January 2022

Published by
Pure Carbon Publishing
an Imprint of Living Your Dream, LLC
Glendale, AZ
www.purecarbonpublishing.com

ISBN 13: 978-0-9676887-4-9
Library of Congress Control Number: 2021948695

Edited and Designed by The Story Laboratory
Editor: Kelly Lydick
Interior Design: Tabitha Lahr
www.writeeditdesignlab.com
Author photo by Sharon Langford

This book is dedicated to my dear and loving friend Leslie A. Walling,
who, with encouragement and supreme generosity,
gave me the opportunity to make this happen.

Table of Contents

Tables

Figures

Notes

Introduction

Our preference for cause-and-effect view of body function is a result of what [Arthur] Koestler [1905-1983] has called 'the greatest superstition of our age'—the materialistic clockwork universe of early nineteenth-century physics.

—Larry Dossey, M.D.[1]

This book was written to help find a common understanding between the relatively new analytical sciences, specifically modern physics, modern medicine, and Western herbal medicine and the ancient traditional Eastern herbal medicines.

Herein, I plan to demonstrate the value of ancient Eastern herbal medicines (specifically Ayurveda and Chinese Medicine) by illustrating how its foundations are based on the same sophisticated theories that modern physics has recently rediscovered in the twentieth century.

Because Eastern medicines are phrased in metaphorical language, the descriptions of the effects of herbs and their uses are often difficult and daunting for the analytical Western mindset. This book is to reveal that the problem-solving systems methods of Eastern medicine are comparable to modern physics both of which are phrased in the poetry of our everyday experiences; and thereby bring the valuable field of traditional Eastern herbal medicines into the mainstream of health care.

* * *

When studying science in grammar school, I found it to be very reassuring because it explained the chaotic world around me in very definite terms, which made me feel safe. It is perhaps the reason why I love science and mathematics. But I have since found that living life is not so easily defined and not everybody agrees with the descriptions, such as in the theory of evolution, despite the scientific evidence. In addition, even friends and family members do not always agree with each other's point of view. Life is much more subjective than I had hoped it to be as an idealistic youngster looking for definitive answers.

Notes

Fortunately, the field of modern physics has explained the discrepancies in terms that, not only make sense to me, but at a deep level, I know them to be true from having experienced over six decades of life. In addition, I am glad to know that there are differences of opinion or life would be very boring. Indeed, modern physics shows how interesting life can be. Therefore, in the following pages are some of the concepts I have found to be true, at least from my *relative* perspective.

Having been trained in the hard sciences, I truly enjoy learning about modern physics, especially its profound concepts and implications. The more I learned, the more I realized how much modern physics was like Eastern medicine and more parallels came to light.

Before ever hearing of the physicist Fritjof Capra and his ground-breaking book *The Tao of Physics*, I was writing about the parallels between modern physics and Eastern medicine and thinking that I was the only person who had seen the parallels between the two fields. When I was finally introduced to his books, I found information on the concepts of modern physics that I had been looking for and, therefore, I have quoted extensively from Fritjof Capra's books here. While Dr. Capra's insights begin from the viewpoint of modern physics, my viewpoint arrives at the same conclusions but from the perspective of Eastern medicine.

A pivotal episode in my life was a car accident in 1988 where I fractured my back and leg. I was hospitalized for a month and took nine months to physically recover. I am grateful to Western medicine for their ability to fix things that are physically broken. However, in my healing process, I rejected the pain drugs instinctively knowing they were detrimental to my body-mind healing. This experience gave me a lot of time to think about what was important to me, which is helping others to heal. That realization propelled me back into studying herbal medicine.

Since the age of five I have been aware of an 'inspirational connection" inside me. That's where my multi-dimensional systems-thinking comes from. It is probably why I have been able to professionally and successfully work at different disciplines such as: archaeology, assistant curator of the Phoenix Art Museum, geologist, studying classical ballet, organic gardening, festival creator and organizer, and, more recently, poetry.

Even though I grew up on the concrete sidewalks of Brooklyn, New York, I have always loved Nature's plants and animals. Most of my poetry is inspired by my love of nature, but so is my work in Eastern medicine. Because I love that animals are so honest, unselfconscious, and unconditionally accepting, I also work with my many animals (cats, dogs, horses, goats, chickens) using Eastern medicines.

As a practitioner of Eastern herbal medicine since 1994, I have a deep understanding of problem-solving systems-thinking. Since 1974, herbal medicine has been my passion. I originally practiced Western herbal medicine but was disenchanted because I could see the results were inconsistent and its application symptomatically haphazard, so I stopped practicing for several years as I found it unsatisfying.

Then, in a lecture by Deepak Chopra, I was introduced to Ayurveda and knew instantly that Ayurveda had the missing pieces my scientific-poetic mind was looking for. Soon after, I found the Ayurvedic Institute in Albuquerque, New Mexico and regularly travelled there for years to study with Dr. Vasant Lad, an Ayurvedic physician. From Dr. Lad I learned what I innately knew—that science is poetry.

At the same time, I was studying Ayurveda, I studied with Michael Tierra, L.Ac., and began learning Chinese Medicine. This may sound daunting to some, but for me, it was wonderful to discover the parallels between the two modalities. Here was another field of study that seemed to have no restrictions on multi-dimensional systems-thinking. So, it was natural for me to see the parallels between the two ancient medicines and then correlate them with modern physics where systems-thinking is also acknowledged.

As physicist Amit Goswami says,

> *Until recently, scientists have been much too carried away with emphasizing the rational and continuous processes of scientific investigation. But creativity is nonrational and discontinuous. And science involves creativity in a major way.*[2]

So, let's get creative!

Notes

Part One:

Old & New Paradigms

Notes

Chapter 1:

Ancient But Not Obsolete

It is more important to have beauty in one's equations than to have them fit experiment.

—Paul Dirac, physicist[1]

Many systems of medicine have been passed down to us through millennia; the oldest being Ayurveda, Chinese, Greek, Unani, and Native American medicines. All these health promoting systems have herbal medicine in common and have been practiced for thousands of years. The longevity of these forms of medicine means that they are available to us because they continue to be effective. In contrast, Western medicine is about 170 years old beginning with the publication of Robert Remak's (1815-1865) discovery of cellular pathology.

Each ancient system of herbal medicine has its strong points but the oldest of herbal medicines, Ayurveda and Chinese Medicine, have the most explicit documented uses, methods, and results. This is evidenced by their extensive materia medicas or "healing materials," system-based theories paralleling modern physics, and their longevity of existence due to their effectiveness.

The Theory of Humors

The Theory of Humors (a system of governing principles in bodily health) was made popular in ancient Greece by Galen (131-201 AD). The Theory of Humors was used until it was displaced in 1855 by Rudolf Virchow's (1821-1902) publication of Robert Remak's discovery of cellular pathology stating that all cells originate from existing cells.

The theory of cellular pathology was an important step forward in understanding the structural biology of living things. However, the resultant abandoning of the functioning system of Theory of Humors was like "throwing the baby out with the bathwater" changing medicine from systems-thinking to linear-thinking (See Chapter 2).

Notes

The Theory of Humors first appeared in Ayurveda over 5,000 years ago. Humors encompass our physical, mental-emotional, and spiritual tendencies and explain our innate constitution. Humors also apply to the different qualities of the disorders that affect our bodies. It is a metaphorical or poetic way of describing the processes of our internal environmental conditions—hot, cold, wet, dry, (Chapter 4) and Nature's Five Phases of Space, Air, Fire, Water, Earth and their combinations (Chapter 5). These conditions and Phases are reflected in, and affect, the internal systems and processes of our bodies. They also affect our environment since we are made up of the same materials.

The Five Phases are present in our bodies in differing proportions, depending on a person's unique constitution and presenting disorder or condition. This is analogous to the environment which exhibits general climates, similar to body constitutions, (See Chapter 11) and variations of weather or conditions within the climate.

The Theory of Humors also explains the different mental-emotional, and spiritual tendencies and, therefore, the attributes of people who possess different combinations of the Five Phases of Space, Air, Fire, Water, and Earth. For example, the classical Greeks would say someone is phlegmatic when discussing a person who tends to be laid-back and tolerant—from the qualities of the Water Phase; melancholic when a person is serious and moody—from qualities of the Earth Phase; sanguine when a person is sociable and optimistic—from qualities of the Air Phase; choleric when a person is extroverted and aggressive—from qualities of the Fire Phase; and spacey when a person is not focused—from the qualities of the Space Phase. These effects occur because of the influence of The Five Phases on our mental-emotional states. This will be discussed in more detail in Chapter 5.

According to the Theory of Humors, disease was caused by any one Phase or combination of The Five Phases when they accumulated in the body. To bring the body back into its dynamic-balance or health, the ancient herbal practitioner would reduce the accumulated condition by using herbal medicine. That is, if one had too much heat (Fire Phase) such as fever, the protocol would be to reduce the hot-fever condition; if one was too cold with a lot of mucus (Air and Water Phases) the method would be to increase heat (Fire Phase) in the body to dry the mucus (Water Phase) and warm the person.

Also, important, the herbs used would be dependent on the constitution (Humor) of the person so as not to further imbalance the person or create side-effects. Side-effects occur when the treatment does not allow for the context of the person, a systems concept that is determined by The Functional Principles Theory.

The Functional Principles Theory and The Theory of Relativity

Ancient traditional herbal medicines are founded on the theory of Functional Principles (also known as Energetics). *The Functional Principles Theory is the process of classifying herbal medicine according to the effects of the different combinations of The Five Phases*; or, using Nature as a metaphor, *to classify the actions and experiential effects of The Five Phases of Matter on the context of mind, body, and consciousness to describe biological and scientific processes and principles.*

In other words, the theory of The Functional Principles is the theories of modern physics that also uses metaphoric poetic terminology to describe our world and experiences.

Underlying all ancient medicine is the understanding of the physics of energy-matter, and before that, the Awareness (discussed in Chapter 7) that perceives energy-matter. The ancients knew the difference between energy and matter is simply a matter of space. Modern physics confirms there is merely more relative space in energy than there is in matter. They are the same substance in a different phase of expression like ice (solid), water (liquid), and steam (air).

On the surface, it appears each modality of ancient herbal medicine has different principles—Yin and Yang, Doshas, Humors—for context-applied herbal medicine. But essentially, the foundation of all ancient herbal medicines is the dynamic systems-method of The Functional Principles based on the understanding of the Theory of Relativity and modern physics.

The Theory of Relativity & Modern Physics

The Theory of Special Relativity, published in 1905 by Albert Einstein, states that, "Two events, simultaneous for one observer, may not be simultaneous for another observer if the observers are in relative motion." [2] Therefore, the relationship of mass, or substance, and energy, in the above scenario, depends on the frame of reference of the observer; which means that from where you stand things look different from where I stand.

Through physics experiments in the 1920s, physicists demonstrated that our awareness influences the matter or objects we perceive. ". . . once a measurement is done, the measured system becomes entangled with *both* the physicist who measured it *and* a huge number of other particles. . . "[3] Therefore, our unique or individual relative perception influences the things we observe; or, with our unique awareness we influence and determine what we choose to see—and so objectivity is an illusion.

Despite this profound scientific insight into our existence, Western culture is held captive by materialism that recognizes only one aspect of our lives—material substance and quantifiable data—as the only acceptable reality. The significance of our experiences (the value of context) is not acknowledged or considered valid because our individual experiences and perceptions cannot be scientifically proven or measured.

Most of us intrinsically know that the numbers tell only a small part of our story. Therefore, understanding the non-linear process-method of The Functional Principles system, offers us valuable insight into not only our health but our relationships, career choices, community, institutions, and governments. That insight, can provide for positive and balanced change in our lives and culture once we let go of illusory materialism. Fritjof Capra in his book, *The Tao of Physics,* states the same conclusion:

> *Thus, the awareness of the profound harmony between the world view of modern physics and the views of Eastern [medicine] now appears as an integral part of a much larger cultural transformation, leading to the emergence of a new vision of reality that will require a fundamental change in our thoughts, perceptions, and values.*[4]

Notes

Notes

Ayurveda

Ayurveda (see Chapter 7) is the oldest system of medicine dating from over 5,000 years ago. Every ancient practice of herbal medicine uses some aspect of the Theory of Humors that first appeared in Ayurveda. Ayurveda is believed to have originated in northern India, where it is still practiced today. The knowledge and wisdom of Ayurveda then spread from India throughout the Orient and eventually to the Western world.

Ayurveda's system of herbal medicine classification has its foundation in The Five Phases (Chapter 5) demonstrating the experiential effects of energy and matter in Nature. The Vedic sutras poetically describe effects of energy-matter in Ayurvedic medicine, which have subsequently been revealed by the Theory of Relativity and modern physics, to show that ". . . the classical ideal of an objective [mechanistic] description of nature is no longer valid."[5] Modern physics experiments prove we are part of, not separate from Nature; we participate in and create our world.

From the Five Phases of Space, Air, Fire, Water, and Earth, emerged the concept of *The Functional Principles Theory— the classification of herbal medicine according to the effects of the different combinations of The Five Phases; or the scientific laws of physics, demonstrated by the actions and experiential effects of The Five Phases of Matter on the context of mind, body, and consciousness to describe biological and scientific processes and principles.*

The Functional Principles Theory is the foundation of the profound science and poetry of Ayurveda, and its derivatives. It is because these ancient forms of medicine merged the science of physics and reality of experience that they have continued their remarkable effectiveness and longevity.

Chinese Medicine

Chinese Medicine (see Chapter 8) is between 3,000-4,000 years old and is also based on The Five Phases (in Chinese Medicine some of the terminology differs) and, also, therefore, the science of modern physics and poetry of experience. From the observation of the effects of the qualities of The Five Phases on mind-emotions, spirit, and physical matter, came the profound theory of Yin and Yang or the duality and relativity of Nature.

The Theory of Relativity states that the relationship of mass and energy depends on the frame of reference of the observer. Using Chinese Medicine, where mass is the Yin and energy is the Yang, then the observer is the interrelationship between the two. Chinese Medicine based its principles and medicine, over three thousand years ago, on Yin and Yang, the theory of the inherent duality and the interdependence and relativity of Nature.

Greek, Unani, Native American

Though we will not be discussing Greek, Unani, and Native American herbal medicine in any detail, suffice it to say they also have their beginnings in the concepts of The Five Phases and The Functional Principles Theory as can be seen by the similar concepts noted below. (See Table 1.1.)

There is a fundamental difference between the Eastern theories of Ayurveda and Chinese Medicine and Greek-derived medicine of which Western medicine is an example. Although its basis was energetic, it is from classical Greek philosophy that the mechanistic, linear theory of the universe of Euclidian geometry evolved and on which we have based our Western culture and medicine. Greek medicine and its derivatives are "non-relativistic."[6]

Greek and Unani medicines are founded on the concept of the four Humors—Blood, Phlegm, Yellow Bile, and Black Bile—to describe different bodily constitutions (context).

Native American medicine uses the four directions, set in a wheel, to describe the effects of herbs—north, east, south, and west that are similar to The Five Phases.

Notes

Table–1-1

TRADITIONAL MEDICINES

Humors, Experience, Phases

CHINESE MEDICINE			AYURVEDA		
YIN-YANG-QI	EXPERIENCE	PHASE	DOSHA	EXPERIENCE	PHASE
Qi	Mobile & Hot	Air & Fire	Vata	Mobile & Cold	Air & Space
Yang	Hot	Fire	Pitta	Hot	Fire & Water
Yin	Wet & Cold	Water & Earth	Kapha	Wet & Cold	Water & Earth

UNANI			NATIVE AMERICAN		
HUMOR	EXPERIENCE	PHASE	DIRECTION	EXPERIENCE	PHASE
Blood	Hot & Moist	Fire & Water	East	Hot	Fire
Phlegm	Cold & Moist	Space & Water	South	Cold & Moist	Water
Yellow Bile	Hot & Dry	Fire & Space	West	Heavy & Static	Earth
Black Bile	Cold & Dry	Space & Air	North	Mobile & Cold	Air
			Center	Cold & Dry	Space

Notes

Chapter 2:

Linear & Systems Thinking

. . . The structures and phenomena we observe in nature are nothing but creations of our measuring and categorizing mind.

—Fritjof Capra, physicist[1]

Linear Thought

Nature is non-linear. Nature, a living system, is composed of processes with small and seemingly chaotic variables that make precise predictions impossible. The classical mathematical equations that scientists have established to describe Nature's complex processes have left out these small variables, so equations can be solved analytically with definitive numerical answers. Unfortunately, scientists eventually came to believe their equations were accurate descriptions of Nature, hence our linear and mechanical or Cartesian science, thought, social institutions, and culture.[2]

In linear equations, small changes will show small effects and large changes will show large effects. However, in non-linear or in the systems of natural phenomena, there exist self-regulatory processes, called feedback loops, that can produce significantly large effects with small changes. Feedback loops take the output of a system and use that output to adjust the natural system to meet a desired response that can be vastly different than the original output. The natural system learns by using these feedback loops.

More recently, scientists have discovered that Nature's apparent chaos is a profound and complex intelligent non-linear system. In other words, the influence of the many factors in ecological systems can be generalized but not accurately predicted.

For example, reintroducing the top predator, such as the grey wolf, in an ecosystem has direct effects on the behavior of the prey species, such as the elk. However, the significant indirect effects of reintroducing the wolf, besides the behavior of the elk, could not have been predicted. An example is the regrowth of plant species on hillsides and riparian areas that, in turn, changed the course of the river in Yellowstone National Park. This prey-to-predator feedback loop is called a trophic cascade.[3]

Therefore, what we were taught to believe were simple explanations of Nature's phenomena have turned out to be far more complex than we could ever have imagined. It is, for example, why we are still unable to predict the weather. We understand the linear and mechanistic scientific theories behind the forces that direct the weather, but we are unable to predict the complex feedback loops that create the convoluted patterns that drive the weather.

It is also why, according to physicist Fritjof Capra, that due to the mechanistic biomedical model approach to Western-derived medicines that,

> *. . . modern medicine often loses sight of the patient as a human being, and by reducing health to mechanical functioning, it is no longer able to deal with the phenomenon of healing.*[4]

Notes

Systems Thinking

> *. . . he that breaks a thing to find out what it is has left the path of wisdom.*
>
> —J.R.R. Tolkien, *The Lord of the Rings*[5]

A system is an integrated whole whose unique properties arise from the relationship of its parts. The systems-thinker has been trained in *how* to think, not what to think. A systems-thinker is a problem-solver who comes to understand things systemically by putting them into their context. This approach establishes the nature of their relationships as opposed to just understanding their chemical and functional parts. The properties of the system are the properties of the whole that the smaller parts do not have. If the system is dissected, the properties are subsequently destroyed.

> *. . . material science, is indispensable to the intelligent discussion of . . . material aspects . . . But such knowledge is not necessarily a part of the higher realization of truth. Not only in the realms of life but even in the world of physical energy the sum of two or more things is very often something MORE than, or something DIFFERENT from, the predictable additive consequences of such unions. The entire science of mathematics, the whole domain of philosophy, the highest physics of chemistry, could not predict or know that the union of two gaseous Hydrogen atoms with one gaseous Oxygen atom would result in a new . . . substance— liquid water.*[6]

That is, believing that the numbers from laboratory tests provide us with an indication of health is to assume that reading random, isolated, and individual musical notes will tell

Notes

you what symphony is playing. Indeed, your health may be made up of those numbers, as people makeup members of a family, but they are only parts of the whole; the individuals are not the family.

Science and Poetry

There is motion
But no moving objects.
There is activity
But there are no actors.
There are no dancers,
There is only the dance.
—Fritjof Capra, physicist[7]

The origin of ancient herbal medicines is rooted in what is now called modern physics that is non-linear in its approach. While the language used is not of modern science, its understanding of thermodynamics (the branch of physics that deals with the relationships between heat and energy) and modern physics (the science of the nature and behavior of matter and energy on the atomic and subatomic level)—is profound.

The ancients knew heat moves upward, water seeks its own level, and some diseases can be transmitted by air. They did not need complicated words like thermal units, specific gravity, or the names of certain bacteria or viruses for their methods to work. The evidence of what they knew from systematic observation was apparent all around them provided by Nature herself.

The ancients described their world with imagery and metaphors and with words they used every day such as air, wind, fire, water, earth, heavy, light, hot, cold etcetera, to describe biologic and scientific processes and principles. These words have an experiential meaning more than the scientific terms used to describe them. For example, if we say, "the water is hot enough to burn the skin," we do not need to mention the degrees Fahrenheit to know what is meant. With the experiential words of poetry, we don't need to analyze what is intended by the words. Poetry conveys to us "the heart of matter." With imagery, we can experience it intimately, though vicariously, in our bodies.

Many expressions we use daily are poetic ways of describing what we know to be true of our existence. Most of these expressions refer to our personal experience with and in our bodies. Expressions such as, "that makes me sick to my stomach," when discussing a revolting idea, or "tasty" to describe something pleasing. Think of the poetry in the songs you love or in the prayers that help you get through the day and how they affect your experience.

Poetry allows us to transcend the linear symbols of language. Poetry speaks to us with imagery, the language of the right brain garbed in word-symbols for the benefit of the data driven left brain. Poetry provides understanding through the experience of feeling and sensation, not only through the accumulation of data. Poetry allows us to own an experience as if it happened to us personally. Poetry helps us move away from material facts to what we intrinsically value, experience.

Candice Pert, a pharmacologist, in the 1980s discovered that peptides, short-chain amino acids, are the "biochemical manifestation of emotions..." Peptides form a psycho-emotional network of communication throughout the many non-linear systems of the body. We literally experience our thoughts and emotions with our bodies.[8] Peptides are biochemical expressions of the poetry of the body/mind functioning system.

Limited mechanistic thought assumes only their complicated materialistic language is valid to explain elementary concepts even children understand by experiencing life. Robert Johnson in his essay "Ninety-Six Words for Love" states, "Where there is no terminology, there is no consciousness. A poverty-stricken vocabulary is an immediate admission that the subject is inferior or depreciated in that society."[9] Larry Dossey, M.D. states:

> *It is a common almost uniform, mistake to assume that science can resolve for us what is meant by "real." It is unsettling to discover that modern physical scientists no longer make any claim to reality, . . . The quest for reality is an antiquated one in modern science, belonging to an era that ended with the advent of this century [20th century].*[10]

The statement of facts does not equal our reality. "The direct experience of reality transcends the realm of thought and language. . . "[11] Therefore, reality defines materialistic facts by giving the facts a measure of value and therefore meaning to our experience. In summation:

> *The "scientific method" is merely an intellectual yardstick wherewith to measure material adventures and physical achievements. But being material and wholly intellectual, it is utterly useless in the evaluation of spiritual realities and . . . experience."*[12]

Fact and Context

> *. . . science has been affected by a point of view which tries to be value-free. This is of course mere prejudice.*
>
> —David Bohm, physicist[13]

Ancient herbal medicines embrace the new understanding of modern physics and science to explain the rationale of their theory of Humors and Phases. In contrast, a simplistic mechanistic view has influenced our Western way of thinking and functioning to the present. This simplistic approach allows for data (facts) to be more significant than the person from whom the data was collected, such as in blood tests.

Data is the old language of matter. Data gives us knowledge of the inert part or structure of some object. For example: an arrow has just been shot from a bow. Science can measure the action of the arrow; science can measure the arrow itself, but science cannot measure *why* the arrow was shot from the bow. Was the arrow shot to hit an inanimate target or was it shot to kill? If it was to kill, does it matter if it was in self-defense or cold blood?

The arrow is an object and is measurable matter. The physical action itself can also be measured. But the awareness, the context, cannot be measured but it does give meaning, a value, to the action and the object.

Notes

Notes

Value-determining awareness is discounted in our currently materialistic society because it is relative, unmeasurable, and different for each person. The all-important context-person changes the meaning of the scenario from meaningless, callous fact to a profound significance that affects us deeply. It touches us at the level of experience where we live and what we value. Context defines the value of our reality.

Knowledge Versus Knowing

The direct experience of reality transcends the realm of thought and language. . .

—Fritjof Capra, physicist[14]

Knowledge-data and experienced-based-knowing are very dissimilar concepts. Knowledge or data can be obtained by study of the mechanistic parts of matter—one part of our existence devoid of the value of experience.

Knowing is a process obtained by individual experience founded on and then combined with facts—a meaningful and value-oriented description of our reality.

Knowledge results in theories that can be quantified, a linear and limited science. Knowing results in visceral understanding, having no means of measurement. It is therefore an art, like poetry, like life, value oriented.

Together knowledge and knowing, fact and context, science and poetry provide the unity of our reality. Knowing gives value to our knowledge.

* * *

These concepts are what modern physicists have discovered to be reality. It is called the "systems view of life." It is what Eastern medicines are based on.

Notes

Chapter 3:

Linear Medicine

. . . when measure is identified with the very essence of reality, this is illusion.

—David Bohm, physicist[1]

Note: In this and the following chapters we will be discussing and comparing the theories behind ancient Eastern medicines and Western medicine. The purpose is not to discredit or criticize but provide a contrast between Western mechanistic, linear thinking and Eastern systems or problem-solving thinking. As Ted Kaptchuk says: ". . . because Chinese and Western medicine exist simultaneously, and because their philosophies and methods are so different, they provide implicit criticism of each other."[2]

Symptom and Cause in Medicine

The era of modern medicine began with Edward Jenner's discovery of the smallpox vaccine at the end of the 18th century (inspired by the method of inoculation earlier practiced in Constantinople by a Greek woman about 1660 and also in Asia and north Africa called variolation); followed by the discovery of the transmission of disease by bacteria by Robert Koch around 1880 and then his discovery of antibiotics in 1928.

Because of its mechanistic and linear approach, Western medicine, and all medicines derived from Western mechanistic medicine, treats physical symptoms. It is precisely this approach that makes it exemplary in trauma medicine. In other words, if you have a broken leg, the symptomatic treatment is to repair the leg. The person's subsequent response to their broken leg is never addressed, nor should it be at that time.

Notes

However, there is no difference between the cause of a symptom and the response of the intelligent-system that may involve many feedback loops. Western trauma-based medicine treats the symptom—the broken leg, the physical structure; but providing for the intelligent response—the psychosomatic (mind/body) perception of the trauma, that can affect the healing process which then becomes an integral part of the cause—is not addressed. Therefore, not all physical changes in the body are acts of choice, as in accidents, but these imposed physical changes create other structural changes that *are* the result of an intelligent system.[3]

According to the Santiago Theory of Cognition by Humberto Maturana and Francisco Varela, living beings first perceive and then respond (as opposed to react) at many different levels of their being.[4] The responses vary from individual to individual and can be physical as well as emotional which then have other effects in the living system, such as post-traumatic stress syndrome. In Western medicine, the consequent response is ignored so the immediate trauma can be remedied, which is a good thing at the time of physical trauma.

Figure–1

REACTION VS. RESPONSE

Reaction-Symptom | **Response-Pattern**

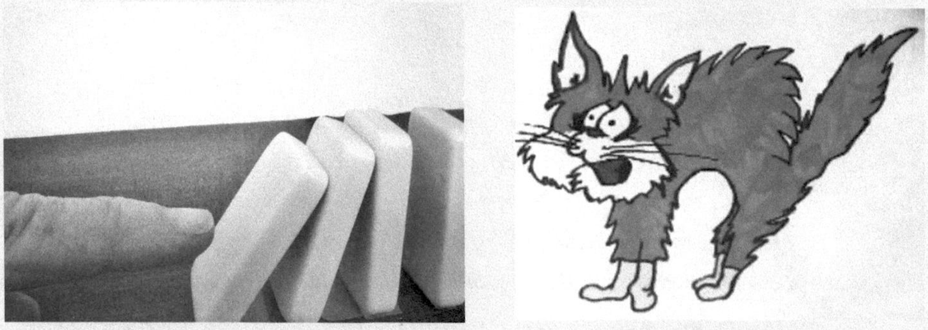

In reaction-symptom, the cause is the finger pushing the panels with the reaction being, the panels fall over—a matter of physics. In response-pattern, something that scared the cat caused a surge of adrenaline; its intelligent response is its hair standing on end. The fright response (adrenaline) and cause (adrenaline) are the same.

Artwork by Sharon Langford

In Eastern medicine, once the physical trauma is treated, the psychosomatic (mind/body) response-pattern becomes the consequent root-cause that, in turn, may become a chronic condition. The original impetus was the broken leg but the subsequent psychosomatic response-pattern, or feedback loops, have now created an imbalanced system with, for example, symptoms of long-term chronic pain. Therefore, the psychosomatic root-cause—the chronic pain response-pattern, and the subsequent long-term chronic pain effect—also the response-pattern, is the same.

The root-cause can also be what Western medicine eventually labels a disease or an ailment. Every constitution, or living intelligent system, has its own unique response-pattern to a trigger. It is why in Eastern medicine we treat each person's response-pattern to the same root-cause differently. Western medicine simply treats the disease or ailment irrespective of the person's unique response-pattern or context.

According to modern physics and Nobel Prize winning physicist Werner Heisenberg's (1901-1976) uncertainty principle (published 1927), causality in quantum physics does not exist; there is a randomness to nature's essence.[5] Therefore, the response pattern of an intelligent system is unpredictable and varied, probabilistic in nature—what is called nonlocal in modern physics. This would account for why people with the same ailment or injury respond differently. It is a concept on which Eastern medicine is founded.

The Eastern medicine practitioner wants to know *why* and *how* your response-pattern was a headache as opposed to another possible response. If the stimulus was stress, the headache would be treated differently from a sinus headache, or one due to dehydration. The response-pattern varies in different disorders and in different people which is why context is so important.

The goal of Eastern medicine is to assist and guide the body back into its innate and dynamic balance, or positive feedback loops; and to undo the negative-acting feedback loops, so the disorder is unlikely to reappear.

Physicist David Bohm explained in speaking of a stream described exactly how Eastern medicine approaches disease.

> *Rather, we will look at the whole situation, and be attentive and alert to learn about it, and thus to discover what is really an appropriate sort of action, relevant to this whole, for bringing the. . . [negative-acting feedback loops] to an end.*[6]

According to biologist Ludwig von Bertalanffy (1901-1972), living systems function with a "flowing balance." That is, in living systems the structure is relatively stable but within it there is a constant flow of energy and matter.[7] The expertise of the Eastern medicine practitioner is restoring this essential flow of energy and substances in the body/mind-systems so the intelligence of the body/mind can re-establish its own unique flowing-balance or innate positive-acting feedback loops.

The systems-thinking, problem-solving Eastern medicine practitioner will ask many questions and use various diagnostic tools to determine the *response-pattern* of the body/mind system. The symptoms will then form a *pattern of imbalance*, or pattern of negative-effecting feedback loops, that point to the correct treatment strategy to eliminate the root-cause or undesired system-response. Another way of saying this is, the Eastern medicine practitioner wants to know the *relationships* between the disorder and the person to be treated.

The body, as Capra states, is composed of ". . . dynamic patterns which do not exist as isolated entities, but as integral parts of an inseparable network of interactions."[8] Therefore, the Eastern practitioner must understand and perceive the entire self-regulating, process-oriented, and network-functioning microcosm of the body/mind to make sense of the pattern, or feedback loops, that is labeled a disease or disorder. Eastern medicine has understood this multi-dimensional, non-linear concept of the body/mind for many millennia.

Notes

Notes

Linear-Mechanistic Thinking and Its Medicines

> *There is a growing awareness among them [physicians] that many of the problems our medical system faces stem from the reductionist [mechanistic] model of the human organism on which it is based.*
>
> —Fritjof Capra, physicist[9]

Western Medicine

In the first decade of the twentieth century, medical education became focused on biochemistry and physiology to the exclusion of the sciences that deal with human nature such as, philosophy, sociology, and epidemiology (the study of the origin, distribution, and control of disease).[10] "The drive to improve medical cure to the neglect of medicine care carried the day."[11] All other forms of medicine were discredited and eventually eliminated as being invalid. Schools other than Western medicine were eliminated by 1938 and eventually deemed illegal. The American Medical Association (AMA) with support from the wealthy, financially biased Rockefeller General Education Board, Carnegie and other foundations, was able to make the AMA the exclusive authority on medicine based on the outdated mechanistic view of the universe and life.[12] Ironically, this unfortunate mechanistic domination of the former systems-based medicine thwarted Western medicine's ability to evolve for the populous, and was occurring at the same time that the liberating Theory of Relativity and Quantum Physics were being developed.

The monopoly of the AMA eliminated all forms of other medicines, and promoted Western medicine based on expensive pharmaceutical drugs. The subsequent discovery of penicillin and other "miracle" drugs convinced the public of the efficacy of Western medicine to the exclusion of all others.

These errors are also due to Western medicine's assumption that by dissecting a body or living system we could understand how it works. Studying the parts of a body does not give us the understanding of the whole pattern that identifies the individual being studied. As Capra states:

> *Systemic properties are properties of a pattern. What is destroyed when a living organism is dissected is its pattern. The components are still there, but the configuration of relationships among them—the pattern—is destroyed, and thus the organism dies.*[13]

In other words, Western medicine has based its suppositions of diagnosis and treatment on how lifeless, and often diseased, tissue appears instead of approaching vital health in terms of patterns of connectedness and relationships in the context of the whole person. In fact, the subjects of health, healing, and healthy lifestyles are not topics of learning in medical schools as they are outside the scope of modern medicine.[14]

Western medicine's symptomatic approach can save lives by treating trauma, but it is limited in effectively dealing with the day-to-day illnesses, such as colds and flus, post-trauma healing, and sub-clinical symptoms of malaise that plague man and animal.

Herbal Medicine in History

Notes

Herbal Medicine has been the medicine of necessity and choice from the beginning of history. About 80% of our planet's population still actively uses herbal medicine as its foremost source of health care.

In the distant past, due to fear of the unknown causes of illnesses, the clever and shrewd ancient medicine man used everything from deception to fear in order to gain influence among his people by using mysterious rituals. With this influence, the ancient medicine man could put himself in a place of power and influence.

Ancient people, and some cultures today, believe spirits, magic (evil eye), and sin, caused illness. They had faith in the medicine man's remedies, usually herbal, charms, fetishes, magic, rituals, signs, and omens. The Greeks believed in the efficacy of oracular advice; many cultures used magic as protection against demons. Other cultures used and still use various forms of superstition. The advent of scientific understanding has helped to lessen man's superstitious fear of the mysterious causes of human misery and suffering.

The common people today, still subject to fear and superstition, due to the lack of adequate and proper education, have been misled into allowing this ancient deception to perpetuate, not only in Western medicine, but in our Western institutions. Barbara Griggs in *Green Pharmacy, A History of Herbal Medicine,* explains why:

> *There are a number of obvious reasons for this prejudice. Herbal medicine is damned by association in medical eyes because it belongs to medicine's dark and discreditable past, when doctors were so often ineffectual; because it is practiced by people they consider inadequately trained, if at all; because it is practiced by lay-people trying to doctor themselves; and because it is practiced by peasants and primitive people the world over. There is, moreover, a major communication problem between the orthodox and the herbal practitioner to be overcome, with years of mistrust, suspicion, skepticism or hostility on both sides threatening the possibility of a good working relationship. Much more of the professional prejudice against medicinal herbs comes from ignorance. The Western doctor today grows up in an atmosphere of extreme skepticism about the value of plants in his materia medica—a skepticism which the big drug companies certainly do nothing to dispel.*[15]

It is the continued association of herbal medicine with lingering superstition and lack of adequate and professional training that is offensive to modern science and medicine.[16] Part of the scope of this book is to obliterate this antiquated and largely false association and help to bring into the 21st century and mainstream health care the valuable and professional systems-based Eastern herbal medicine.

Notes

Western Herbal Medicine

Western herbal medicine, though it originally included the process-thinking Greek Theory of Humors, gradually disregarded this foundation and began to focus on the symptomatic uses of herbal medicine. This unfortunate decline began sometime during the 1800s when the roots of modern Western medicine began its "heroic" forms of treatment.

Having shifted to mechanistic thought, Western herbal medicine now lacks a consistent system of treatment and understanding of how to qualify the person-context, and therefore, is also symptomatic in its approach. In addition, the organs of the body are taught as separate units devoid of the vital inter-relationships that bring meaning to the whole person and their condition.

However, the highly trained systems-based herbal medicine practitioner or "Systems Herbalist" (see below for more on Systems Herbalist) would have a comprehensive systems-based foundation to avoid resorting to symptoms and an understanding of how to qualify the person-context, their unique patterns and inter-relationships. This is discussed further in Chapter 12.

The lack of both foundational principles and a clear system for diagnosis encouraging the practice of symptomatic treatment has been a problem throughout medicine's history as early as the Tang-dynasty (3rd to 10th centuries) in China when a physician said:

> *Nowadays people are unable to. . . recognize the origins of disease. They base decisions on their feelings and use many medicinal substances. This is like hunting for rabbits by sending out many men and horses to surround the area in the hope that, by luck, one of them will stumble upon the rabbit. Treating like this is really negligent.*[17]

Today, in its efforts to find a secure foundation, clinical Western herbal medicine has looked to the mechanistic approach of scientific data from research on chemical constituents of herbs or phytochemistry. However, modern physics has found that you cannot understand something by looking at its smaller parts. As Fritjof Capra says,

> *. . . the constituents of matter and the basic phenomena involving them are all interconnected, interrelated and interdependent; they cannot be understood as isolated entities but only as integrated parts of the whole.*[18]

This is also true of herbal medicines where the separate chemical constituents do not give us a consistent indication of what the entire herb is capable of accomplishing. Biochemist, Rupert Sheldrake explains:

> *Attempting to explain organisms in terms of their chemical constituents is rather like trying to understand a computer by grinding it up and analyzing its component elements. Certainly, it is possible to learn something about the computer in this way, namely what it is made of. But this process of reduction, the structure and the programmed*

activity of the computer vanishes, . . . ; no amount of mathematical modelling of interactions between its atomic constituents will reveal the computer's programs or the purposes they fulfilled.[19]

Notes

The concept that parts can only be understood by its relationships with other parts in the context of the whole is called systems-thinking. According to the systems-thinking of 21st century scientists, Capra states,

Living systems [of which herbs are a part] are integrated wholes whose properties cannot be reduced to those of smaller parts. Their essential, or "systemic," properties are properties of the whole, which none of the parts have.[20]

Therefore, as we cannot expect to understand an organism by dissecting it, we also cannot understand the actions of an herb by "dissecting" it into its chemical constituents. The systemic properties or synergistic actions of an herb are destroyed when the herb is isolated into chemical constituents.[21]

A paper in "Pharmacopsychiatry" exemplifies the issue of trying to extract the active ingredient in an herb.

Modern science has tried to identify the active constituents in an herb in order to isolate the chemical responsible for the effect to see if the ingredient could be synthesized, patented, and mass produced. However, it has been found in several cases (so far) where the so-called 'active ingredient' is not what they originally thought it to be. For example, the herb St. John's Wort, Hypericum perforatum, was originally thought to have the substance hypericin as its active ingredient. Then several years later a study was done where they found that not to be the case.[22]

The other extreme is mysticism whose mastery is predicated on years of arduous discipline to transcend the balancing act of mind, matter, and spiritual realities. Mysticism has the system-thinking but has no interest in applying it to the material world as it is considered irrelevant. While these sage experts exist, few are known practicing herbalists.

Systems Herbalist

The new designation of "Systems Herbalist" herein referred to is defined as follows:

A systems-based herbal medicine practitioner or "Systems Herbalist" has an education in medicine, pre-medicine, or the hard sciences, such as biology, chemistry, and anatomy and physiology, and is also educated and well versed in Eastern medicine theory, principles, and systems-thinking.

The Systems Herbalist would also be trained to gather facts from the physical, experiential, and non-physical realms of life, intuition (understanding without the need for

Notes

conscious reasoning) and to accurately assess the "patterns of disharmony" present in a person, without resorting to treating symptoms; and to determine the herbal treatment, food and lifestyle guidelines necessary to help rebalance a person's system based on The Functional Principles Theory as exemplified by Ayurvedic and Chinese Medicine. This will be discussed further in Chapters 7 and 8. According to Albert Einstein, "The only real valuable thing is intuition."

The following is a suggestion for levels of competence for the Systems Herbalist. Anyone who has not had the basic training of the Level I Systems Herbalist is a Folklore Herbalist who continues to be of value to family and friends.

Level I—Systems Herbalist:

- The herbalist who has been in practice a minimum of 1-5 years.
- Has a minimum of 2,300 hours of clinical training and herbal pharmacy training.
- Is proficient in the use of the systems-thinking of Eastern medicine.
- Has earned a four-year undergraduate degree.
- Has studied anatomy, physiology, biology, biochemistry, pharmacology, pathology, botany, basic physics, and counseling.
- Continuing research and education.
- Is focused and dedicated to being of service to their clients. "Fixing and helping may be the work of the ego [but] service [is] the work of the soul."[23]
- Begins and continues a regular meditation/introspection practice to improve focus, memory, mental clarity, and reduce stress.

Level II—Systems Herbalist:

- The herbalist who has been in practice between 5 to 10 years.
- Has met the criteria in Level I.
- Continues in clinic practice for a minimum of 1,000 hours per year.
- Continues ongoing research and education.
- Continues to be focused and dedicated to being of service to their clients.
- Continues a regular meditation/introspection practice.

Level III—Systems Herbalist:

- The herbalist who has been in practice 10+ years.
- Has met the criteria in Level I & II.
- Continues in clinical practice for a minimum of 1,000 hours per year.
- Continuing research and education.
- Continues to be focused and dedicated to being of service to their clients.
- Has learned to integrate social, economic, family, and community into the healing process.
- Has continued a regular meditation/introspection practice.

Part Two:

Traditional Systems of Herbal Medicine

Notes

Chapter 4:

More Than the Sum of Its Parts: Herbs

Herbs
Green physicians
Mighty messengers of life
Rooting their wisdom
Into our bodily turf.

Verdant offerings
Remember us to mend
With gentleness, compassion
Bring us to blossom end.

From seed to flower
All a bouquet of power
To grow the planted memory
Of our nature divinity.
— J. Shamosh

Herbs and Pharmaceutical Drugs

Herbs are organic, life-sustaining foods that stimulate receptors and chemical reactions to influence the body-systems to respond with a less psychosomatically negatively-acting feedback loop than the one that created the undesirable response. In addition, herbs/foods provide the nutrition and energy to support the move toward flowing-balance of a

Notes

healthier systems-response. Consider that herbal medicines are nature's re-programmers of the body-mind connection.

According to physicist, Amit Goswami, that is exactly what happens to the human body when it is ill; its software has gone awry and, due to the destructive patterns of the body-mind, it is unable to cure itself. Further, Goswami states that in order to heal itself the quantum body-mind connection needs to be accessed and repaired so that the body can be reprogrammed to heal itself.[1]

In contrast, pharmaceutical medications are lifeless, foreign, and antagonistic substances to the body—chemical compounds that do not give the system a choice as to how it may respond. As if it were a machine, the body-system is forced to react, as opposed to respond, without the system's intelligent input.

In addition, drugs do not contain nutrients to sustain the body to support the unnatural changes they provoke. These forced changes deplete the body's nutrients and energy resources producing further undesirable reactions that we know as side effects.

Drugs force the body to do things it would not do normally because it is not in the body-system's pattern to respond that way. For example, prednisone forces the body to secrete adrenal hormones without providing the nutritional support to do so. In turn, over time, the body's response-pattern is to steal nutrients from other organs to continue the sham thereby generating undesirable side effects. It is akin to forcing someone to work without providing adequate food, water, and rest.

Drugs appear to short-circuit the peptide based psychosomatic network, discovered by pharmacologist Candice Pert in the 1980s, that connects the nervous, immune, and endocrine systems, disabling, if not damaging, the intelligent communication between them. Therefore, drugs are a poison if used long-term.

From an Eastern medicine perspective, pharmaceutical drugs create a reaction or change in the body without the support of nutrients and energy to maintain the change. This contrasts with a normal response where the entire system participates in a pattern that continually maintains its flowing balance. Eventually the sustained energetic reaction will burn out the supporting substances of the body's systems. Lacking the organic, life-sustaining, and nourishing compounds of herbal medicines is one reason why drugs are so depleting to the body.

The use of pharmaceutical drugs suppresses illness instead of resolving illness. As a result, the illness is driven into the deeper layers of the body where it festers creating unseen insidious havoc only to emerge decades later as a serious disease that is never associated with the original suppressed illness.

In addition, in the dispensing of drugs, doctors are not trained to consider the receiver of the drug and how it may further disrupt the unique pattern and flowing balance of the individual person or context.

Having said the above, drugs do save lives in acute situations. However, continuous use of them is detrimental. Once the system is stabilized, their use should be gradually declined while using herbal remedies, lifestyle changes, and proper diet to support the system to take over the effects of the drugs.

The Eight Experiential Effects

Notes

Eastern herbal medicine uses The Functional Principles Theory to classify herbs according to the Eight Experiential Effects of the different combinations of the Five Phases. That is, Eastern herbal medicine combines the dynamic science of modern physics and science as demonstrated by the actions and experiential effects of The Five Phases (discussed in Chapter 5) on the mind, body, consciousness, and all matter.

The actions of The Five Phases are categorized into Eight Experiential Effects that transmit the chemical actions or potency of the herbs or foods into our bodies.

For example, to treat a condition of Heat and Damp in the lower body we would use herbs/foods that transmit cooling, drying, and downward effects. The heat would be cooled, the damp dried, and the downward effect would target the area of the body to be addressed by using the correct herbal formula that has these properties.

Heating Effect

Heat is a form of energy caused by either the excitation of electrons in atoms, the combination of two substances creating a thermochemical reaction, or a reaction transferring the chemical sensation of heat to another substance; in this case, receptors called nociceptors in the body.[2] Certain herbs/foods can generate this chemical sensation of heat such as capsicum (Capsicum annuum, fruit), that is measured in Scoville units of heat. This effect comes from the Fire Phase (The Five Phases are discussed in Chapter 5).

In the body, the heating effect of certain herbs/food can cause dizziness from uprising heat, thirst from the drying effect of heat, fatigue, sweating that creates internal dryness and therefore more heat, and burning sensations, as well as improve digestion due to the stimulation of excretions, appetite, and metabolism. The Pungent, Sour, and Salty Tastes are heating due to the Fire Phase present.

Cooling Effect

> ***How Cold?***
> *When I woke up this morning*
> *It was very cold.*
> *How cold was it?*
> *It was a freezing,*
> *Sneezing goose-bumpy,*
> *Teeth-chattering,*
> *Can't-get-out-of-bed,*
> *Blanket-over-my-head*
> *Kind of cold*
> —Barclay & Donato[3]

The second law of thermodynamics (the branch of physics that deals with the relationships between heat and energy) states that heat flows naturally from an object at a higher temperature to an object at a lower temperature and heat does not flow in the opposite

Notes

direction without added work. In other words, cooling occurs when heat is transferred from a warmer object to a relatively cooler object. And so, cold reduces thermal energy (heat) in a substance reducing the motion of its atomic particles.

And so, the sensation of coolness comes from the transfer of heat from a substance that is warmer to one less warm. That is, coolness is the lack of heat.

But, in this case, a cooling herb will stimulate the nociceptors triggering the neurochemical response to cold and its subsequent physiological responses, such as contraction. This effect is from the Space and Air Phases. An example of a cooling herb would be peppermint (Mentha spp., leaf).

In the body, the cooling effect of herbs/foods refreshes and promotes tissue firmness because of its cooling, contracting effect.

The Sweet, Bitter, and Astringent Tastes have a cooling effect due to the Air and Space Phases.

Drying Effect

The drying effect can come from the Space and Air Phases, the Fire Phase, or the ability of a substance to absorb moisture from something else as in the Earth Phase.

1. Decreasing blood supply by narrowing the small blood vessels—the Space and Air Phases.
2. Pulling water from the tissues—the Fire and Earth Phases.
3. Coagulating the superficial tissue layers into a crust forming a scab—the Air and Earth Phases.
4. Reducing inflammation—the Space, Air, and Water Phases.

The drying effect in the body reduces mucus and damp (wetness) in the body by absorbing moisture from the tissues. The Pungent, Bitter, Salty, Sour, and Astringent Tastes are drying in different ways according to the predominant Phases present.

The Pungent Taste dries because of its heating effect from the Air and Fire Phases, such as the herb garlic (Allium sativum, bulb). The Bitter Taste dries due to its dispersing and stimulating properties, such as coffee (Coffea arabica, seed) from its Space and Air Phases. The Salty Taste dries due to its Fire and Water Phases. The Sour Taste dries due to its Earth and Fire Phases, such as lemons. The Astringent Taste dries due to its dehydrating ability such as black tea (Camellia sinensis, leaf) from the Air and Earth Phases.

Moistening Effect

The moistening effect comes from the ability of a substance to give up its moisture easily to another substance having less moisture. This is like a warmer substance giving up its heat to a cooler substance. Oatmeal (Avena sativa, seed) has a hydrating effect on the tissues of the body.

Another hydrating effect can be achieved by a substance, such as salt, that absorbs moisture and brings it to the dryer tissues.

The moistening effect in the body will increase water and moisture in the body. The Sweet and Salty Tastes moisten by either giving up their own moisture or by attracting it.

The Sweet Taste, such as in slippery elm (Ulmus rubra, bark) is moistening due to the Water and Earth Phases.

The Salty Taste moistens due to its Fire and Water Phases.

Notes

Upward Effect

The herbs/foods with the Air Phase predominant have an upward effect in the body. The Pungent (Air & Fire) and Bitter (Air & Space), and Astringent (Air & Earth) Tastes help to improve digestion and metabolism, detoxify, and reduce fluid in the body, respectively. Heat also moves upward.

An example of the upward effect is any warming spice, such as cayenne (Capsicum annuum, fruit), that can make your head sweat due to the upward moving heat. The Bitter Taste, such as in hops (Humulus lupulus, fruit) used to make beer, that is cooling; bitter also reduces appetite making us feel lighter. The Astringent Taste, such as in an unripe banana that reduces body fluids making you feel lighter.

Downward Effect

Moisture combined with other substances, such as minerals, will be heavier and tend to move to the bottom of the body due to gravity.

The herbs/foods with the heavier Water and/or Earth Phases predominating have a downward effect in the body. The Sweet (Earth & Water Phases), Salty (Fire & Water Phases), Sour (Fire & Earth) Tastes increase weight in the body by either adding or attracting more moisture.

An example of the downward effect is anything heavy such as animal products (Sweet Taste), or sweets, if eaten in large quantities, can make you feel dull and heavy; or salty foods that can make your body retain water.

Inward Effect

The inward effect comes from the ability of a substance to pull moisture away from something else or triggering a cooling effect creating a contracting inward effect. The inward effect is used to dry and create firmness to tissues.

The herbs/foods having an inward effect have the Earth Phase predominant with Astringent (Air & Earth) and Sour (Fire & Earth) Tastes.

An example of Astringent is an unripe banana making your mouth pucker from its drying property; or Sour, as in lemons, also making your mouth pucker (contract).

Outward Effect

The herbs/foods having an outward dispersing effect are predominant in the Air Phase and have the Pungent (Fire & Air) and Bitter (Air & Space) Tastes. These Tastes use heat or movement to disperse a condition out of the body such as a cold or flu.

Heat relaxes the pores that can open to vent heat out of the body by sweating—Air and Space Phases.

Notes

Examples such as ginger (Zingiber officinale, rhizome) that can be used to warm and produce sweating (Fire and Air) and coffee (Bitter Taste) are mentioned above.

Table–4-1

THE EIGHT EFFECTS/THE FUNCTIONAL PRINCIPLES OF THE SIX TASTES

	SWEET	SOUR	SALTY	PUNGENT	BITTER	ASTRINGENT
COOLING	×				×	×
HEATING		×	×	×		
DRYING		×		×	×	×
MOISTENING	×	×	×			
UPWARD				×	×	×
DOWNWARD	×	×	×			
INWARD		×				×
OUTWARD				×	×	

Table-4.2 can be used to help design a formula for a bodily condition. Most herbs/foods are a combination of mainly two Tastes with one Taste predominating. The Six Tastes are discussed in Chapter 6. It then becomes a matter of knowing the effects of the herbs and combining them in a manner resulting in the effect you are trying to accomplish without unwanted side effects to the individual.

Constructing Herbal Formulas

There is no better rationale for constructing herbal formulas than what Chinese Medicine has provided for us. The ancient formulas are elegantly balanced and very effective if used correctly, that is, used for the condition and the presenting response-pattern of the person-context.

Over thousands of years, Chinese herbal medicine has precisely documented how different combinations of herbs affect the different bodily systems, the condition being treated, the potential side-effects, and the all-important response-pattern of the person-context. Chinese herbal medicine has documented the mutual counteractions, suppressions, antagonisms, and incompatibilities of the herbs in their extensive materia medica.[4] It is an art and science unto itself.

Hierarchy of Ingredients in Herbal Formulas

Notes

There is a specific logic and art to constructing an herbal formula to create a desired effect. In fact, in Chinese herbal medicine, the ingredients of a formula are listed in order of importance not quantity. Here again we see the time-honored value of quality over quantity.

Herbal formulas are designed to guide the body to a better response-pattern. You can think of it as a set of instructions that tell the body to respond in a specific way instead of the undesired way. As Bensky and Barolet say, herbal formulas convey "an important message. The formulas are effective in treating disease precisely because of the nature and composition of their ingredients."[5]

- **Chief Herb:** This herb will have the greatest effect on the condition being treated.[6] For example, if one has a fever the Chief herb will be cooling.

- **Deputy Herb:** This herb will assist the Chief herb in treating the condition by having an effect, perhaps slightly different, on the condition being treated.[7] Using the example of someone with a fever, the Deputy herb can help reduce the fever and/or alleviate a headache along with the fever.

- **Assistant Herb:** This herb reinforces the effects of the Chief and Deputy herbs by treating a less important aspect of the condition. It also corrects any toxicity or harshness of the Chief or Deputy.[8] That is, it prevents possible side effects. In the fever condition, the Assistant herb may be one to prevent stomach upset due to the cold quality of the Chief or Deputy herbs.

- **Envoy Herb:** This herb guides the formula to the area of the body being treated. It also helps to coordinate the effects of the other herbs in the formula.[9] With the fever condition, the Envoy herb will be one to guide the formula to the upper body where the headache is located.

Not every formula will have the entire hierarchy of ingredients because some Chief or Deputy herbs may already have an affinity for a certain body location and so an Envoy herb is not necessary. Also, some formulas may have several herbs of a category depending on the nature or severity of the disorder being treated.

Notes

EXAMPLE OF A CHINESE MEDICINE FORMULATION

***Xie Bai* (Drain the Lungs)**

Dry-fried Cortex Mori Albae Radicis *(chao sang bai pi)*
The **Chief** herb used to drain constrained heat from the Lung-System to stop coughing and wheezing.

Cortex Lycii Radicis *(di gu pi)*
The **Deputy** herb used to clear heat from deficiency.

Honey-fried Radix Glycyrrhizae Uralensis *(zhi gan cao)*
The **Assistant** herb used to protect the Stomach-System from the cold properties of the other herbs.

Nonglutinous rice *(geng mi)*
Another **Assistant** herb used to protect the Stomach-System from the cold properties of the other herbs.

From Bensky and Barolet. *Chinese Herbal Medicine Formulas and Strategies,* p 90.

In addition, many of the sophisticated Chinese herbal formulas can be modified depending on how and where the Systems Herbalist wants to direct the treatment. So, minor herbs can be added or subtracted to treat a specific condition.

Clinically, two traditional formulas can be combined with good results. For example, with a headache due to barometric pressure changes, combining a formula to treat the head pain with a formula to eliminate wind in the Liver-System, that is often part of the pattern of these types of headaches, works extremely well.

Uprising wind and phlegm, presenting with dizziness and sometimes seizures due to excess heat in the Liver-System, can be effectively treated by combining two formulas that treat each condition.

In both above situations, the person gets relief within minutes of administering the formulas with no side effects except feeling noticeably better.

Notes

Chapter 5:

From Energy to Matter: The Five Phases

Physicists have come to see that all their theories of natural phenomena, including the 'laws' they describe, are creations of the human mind.

—Fritjof Capra, physicist[1]

The original term for The Five Phases of Energy-Matter is The Five Elements. The word Element is too static and inert sounding whereas Phases of Energy-Matter is more befitting the mutable nature of the concept. The dictionary defines phase as a "distinct period or stage in a process of change for forming part of something's development," and so the term, phase, is more in line with the dynamic nature of modern physics. Henceforth, the term The Five Phases of Energy-Matter, or simply The Five Phases, will be used instead of The Five Elements.

* * *

The Five Phases describe the qualities of the energetic nature of phenomena intrinsic to all matter. The Theory of The Five Phases, which first appeared in Ayurveda, was a departure from the supernatural and superstitious view of Nature to one based on careful and systematic observation of the dynamic patterns within Nature. It is a theory by which one can attain a systems understanding and poetic experience of the processes of Nature.

The Theory of The Five Phases is an accurate description of Nature that can be supported by modern physics and thermodynamics discussed below. The Five Phases precisely and poetically describes the energetic processes that are inherent in the energy-matter of the cosmos.

The ancients knew that matter and energy are diverse manifestations of the same cosmic reality that could only be described by processes within systems. Subsequently,

Notes

systems-thinking has since been confirmed by modern physics to be more accurate than the construct of linear thinking because patterns of energy, of which our reality is based, are not structurally based. Physicist, Fritjof Capra explains:

> *Subatomic particles are not made of any material stuff; they are patterns of energy. Energy, however, is associated with activity, with processes, and this implies that the nature of subatomic particles is intrinsically dynamic. When we observe them, we never see any substance, nor any fundamental structure. What we observe are dynamic patterns continually changing into one another—a continuous dance of energy.*[2]

The Five Phases of Energy-Matter gives us a system to explain these energetic processes inherent in dynamic energy-matter.

For example, water can exist as liquid—water (Water Phase), a solid—ice (Earth Phase), or a gas—steam (Air Phase). The first law of thermodynamics states that to produce work or transformation, you need to supply heat. It is the principle of potential heat of the Fire Phase from the first law of thermodynamics that transforms the liquid-Water Phase to a gas-Air Phase or a solid-Earth Phase.

The second law of thermodynamics states that energy concentrated in one place will always flow to places of lower concentration. It is the action of the Space Phase or the second law of thermodynamics that imparts the lack of heat (Space Phase) or cold to make solid ice (Earth Phase).

Concerning herbal medicine, the Water Phase gives an herb its moistening and cooling qualities, the Earth Phase its stabilizing and drying qualities, the Air Phase its ability to move something, the Space Phase imparting a cooling and dispersing quality, and the Fire Phase its heat conveying, and matter transforming quality. This will be explained further as each Phase is discussed.

By combining The Five Phases in different ways, the experienced herbalist can create specific actions in the body. For example, to moisten and cool the Lungs due to an infection, an herbal practitioner will administer an herbal formula with herbs having a predominance of the Water and Space Phases, or to break up congestion and coldness in the body, use herbs with Air and Fire Phases.

The Poetry of The Five Phases

Modern physics tells us different forms of matter have different amounts of space between their atoms. For example, ice has less space between its atoms than steam. Ice is a condensed form of water and steam a rarefied form of water. In physics, we call ice a solid form of matter and steam a gaseous form of matter. In other words, water can transform through three phases—air, liquid, and solid.

Experiencing ice tells us it is cold and heavy relative to steam that is hot and lightweight. Physics gives us the ability to measure temperature and weight of ice or steam providing us with data that can be quantified. But, experience, the basis of our understanding and existence, gives us the ability to qualify the data provided by science. Experience is the poetry of our existence combined with the facts of science and data to take on meaning and value.

The experiential process of understanding the nature of energy-matter of The Five Phases begins in the realm of rarefied matter and continues through increasingly denser matter.

Notes

The Space/Ether Phase

The Space Phase is also known as the Ether Phase (not to be confused with the actual chemical element of ether) and implies more than simply rarefied space. As alluded to in Eastern mysticism, the Ether Phase implies subatomic energies and/or forces as yet undiscovered by modern physics. Joseph Selbie explains,

> *Quantum physicists theorize that the background energy—sometimes called* vacuum energy *or* zero point energy*—exists in a quantum* energy field *that is present throughout all of space [Space Phase]. . . . it is a restless quantum energy field that is continuously giving rise to matter.*[3]

The Physics of the Space/Ether Phase

Space is not empty. It is a realm where there is a large amount of space between what little matter is present. This relative emptiness contains, besides sparse amounts of physical particles, the force of gravity and electromagnetic radiation as well as other unknown forces suspected, but undiscovered, by physicists. This is the realm that Fritjof Capra spoke of where patterns of energy and activity are abundant.

In modern physics, the Space Phase can be correlated to astrophysicist Sir Fred Hoyle's (1915-2001) theory of a "creation field" where there is a continuous creation of new matter and energy from "quintessence," meaning fifth element—Ether.

It is also possible that biochemist Rupert Sheldrake's (1942-) morphogenic field theory would be contained in the Ether Phase. The morphogenic field is a vibratory pattern of activity, like quantum and electromagnetic fields, that stores a collective memory for a particular system, such as the development of molecules, cells, tissues, organisms, societies, and minds. By the process of morphic resonance, this transfer of information provides an organism with a source of patterns-of-information or memory, such as instinct or the mass collective memory of humanity.[4] The physicist, David Bohm, also discusses this in the concept of "the flux,"

> *. . . that in intelligent perception, the brain and nervous system respond directly to an order in the universal and unknown flux that cannot be reduced to anything that could be defined in terms of knowable structures.*[5]

This concept is very similar to "the cloud" where we store and retrieve our data. Microsoft defines the cloud: "The cloud is not a physical entity, but instead is a vast network

Notes

of remote servers around the globe which are hooked together and meant to operate as a single ecosystem."[6]

> ***Space***
> *Space is a place where I am cold*
> *Nothing here to warm me.*
> *So light I feel, so easy to move*
> *Nothing here to hold me.*
> *So far I see*
> *Nothing here to bar my eye.*
> *Soon I am no more*
> *Nothing here to breathe me.*
> —J. Shamosh

Most of us have never been in outer-space and indeed we could not exist there without protection and support. However, we can imagine what it would feel like if we were able to experience it.

- The first vicarious experience of outer-space is that it is hard to get enough air due to the *rarefied* atmosphere or, it is an atmosphere with far fewer molecules of air than the one we are familiar with at the surface of our planet.
- Once the problem of getting enough air is solved, the next thing you would notice is the extreme *cold* for which you would need a protective suit.
- Then you discover that it is very easy to move around since there is very little atmosphere (matter) to impede your *movement.*
- There is also relatively little matter to obscure your vision thereby giving you a *clear* view.
- Due to the rarefied atmosphere, Space is also *light-weight* and *subtle* in nature.

By vicariously experiencing Space we have some very important information about its qualities-*rarefied, cold, movement, clear, light,* and *subtle.* (See Table 5.1, The Attributes of The Five Phases) These qualities give us insight into the behavior or expression of matter because matter is mostly made up of Space especially in outer-space. We also know the functioning of our world—microcosm—is the same as the universe—macrocosm; in other words, the processes of Nature, or physics, apply everywhere whether on the surface of the planet or in outer-space.

On a more personal level, the Space Phase is expressed in the empty spaces of the body, such as the intestines, blood vessels, lungs, stomach, and bladder.

The Air Phase

Moving from outer-space towards our planet we encounter the relatively denser atmosphere, or the Air Phase, in which we live.

The Physics

Notes

We have moved from the seemingly passive and rarefied realm of the Space Phase to one of greater density where there is more potential energy inherent in the organization of matter or atoms. There is also increased activity due to the movement of the atoms and molecules of our atmosphere.

> ***Air***
> *Elusive in my hand*
> *Moved away with a puff.*
> *Taken by a big motion*
> *Along with my moisture*
> *Parting me cracked, coarse, chill*
> *Unsettled.*
> —J. Shamosh

Our daily experience of Air tells us it is rarefied compared to "solid" objects but not as rarefied as Space.

- Another way of saying something is less rarefied than Space is to say it is *lightweight.*
- *Movement* is intrinsic to Air. Simply by moving your hand you can easily move Air and create a breeze. When more energy is applied, such as with a fan, the breeze can become *wind.*
- A strong wind would make you feel *cold.*
- A constant wind can *dry* your skin as it does the landscape.
- Dry skin feels *rough* or chapped.
- You are also able to see through Air and so it also has a *clear* quality.
- Air is also *subtle* as compared to the heavier Phases such as Water.

The effects of Air are arrived at by our experiencing its qualities of: *movement, cold, dry, rough, light, clear,* and *subtle.* (See Table 5.1, The Attributes of The Five Phases)

Understanding the qualities of Air comes from our *experience* with it daily. We know we cannot live without air for more than a few minutes as it is the main source of food-energy for our bodies. It is not only the molecules of oxygen, nitrogen and other chemical Phases of Air that sustain us but also the energy in the spaces between the atoms, and in the atoms themselves, that contribute to our existence.

The Air Phase is expressed with bodily movement and the movement of substances, such as food, in and out of the body.

The Fire Phase

Most people can easily describe heat because its effects are not at all subtle. But less obvious is the heat from metabolism, and other transformations that heat facilitates, that are essential to our digestion and bodily warmth.

Notes

The Physics

The first law of Thermodynamics states that energy can be neither created nor destroyed and is also known as the conservation of energy.

According to physics, when two surfaces are in contact (in this case, atoms of the Air Phase) and moving relative to each other, the friction converts this kinetic energy into heat, an attribute of the Fire Phase. In physics, heat is the measurement of electronic activity.

Heat can also be produced from thermochemical reactions (a release of potential energy in atoms or molecular bonds) such as those produced by acids. The thermochemical reactions essential to life are based on acids. Acids are defined in terms of what happens when inert salt compounds are dissolved in water. The water molecules become ionized, that is, separated to form positive hydrogen ions (H+) and negative hydroxide ions (OH-). These ions are no longer water per se, but they impart the quality of fluidity to the Fire Phase.

> ***Fire***
> *Bites my touch*
> *Eats all I give*
> *Dancer of grace*
> *Giver of life*
> *It lights my path.*
> —J. Shamosh

- Our experience with fire tells us it is *hot* to the touch.
- Fire has a *fluid* quality as you watch a flame dance and s*pread.*
- Touching the flame would burn you with a *sharp* pain.
- Fire is *lightweight* as heat always rises.
- It is *clear* in that you can see through it.
- We also use heat for its *drying* effect.

Therefore, the qualities of Fire are—*hot, fluid, sharp, light, clear, drying,* and *spreading.* (See Table 5.1, The Attributes of The Five Phases)

The Fire Phase is important because without heat life as we know it could not exist. The Fire Phase, as heat, is the source of all transformation (chemical and physical reactions) essential to life.

The Water Phase

The qualities of water are easily understood and often taken for granted and therefore, many people, when asked about water, forget to mention that it is wet!

The Physics

The essential parts of an acid are the separated ions of water, hydrogen (H+) and hydroxide (OH). That is, as the Fire Phase transforms, it separates becoming water and inert salt compounds (the Earth Phase). In this thermochemical reaction potential heat is released, condensing matter, leaving the Water Phase colder and denser than the Fire Phase. Cold is merely the relative absence of heat.

Notes

> ***Water***
> *Moisture giver*
> *It chills my touch*
> *And unhurried*
> *Runs through my hand*
> *Protesting containment*
> *By its burden.*
> —J. Shamosh

- The most obvious experience with Water is its *wet* quality.
- It feels *cold* to our touch.
- If you tried to lift a quantity of water, it would be *heavy*.
- Water tends to move in a *slow* manner unless activated by something else such as wind.
- It is *dull* as opposed to sharp.
- It moves in a *fluid* manner.

From experience, we know the attributes of Water are—*wet, cold, heavy, slow, dull,* and *fluid.* (See Table 5.1, The Attributes of The Five Phases)

Water is essential to life. Our bodies are 60 percent Water and our planet is 71 percent water. Water moistens our bodies and dissolves and carries nutrients in our bloodstreams to nourish us.

The Earth Phase

The Earth Phase attributes are often taken for granted unless one is a gardener.

The Physics

The thermochemical reaction that produced water also produced inert salts. These inert salts represent the Earth Phase that is denser and colder than the Water Phase. Increased density and coldness in matter is due to less space in the molecular structure and relatively slower atomic motion.

> ***Earth***
> *Unmoving*
> *Arduous*
> *Intense*
> *Chill*
> *Dependable*
> *And oh so loving.*
> —J. Shamosh

Notes

- When lifting a quantity of Earth, we find it to be *heavy*.
- It is *dense*.
- It is *solid*.
- Earth is *cold* to the touch since, by itself, it has no heat.
- Once Earth is put in place it tends to stay there and remains *static*.
- Earth has a *drying* effect your skin.
- Earth contains all the mineral nutrients necessary for the building blocks of plant and body structures, and so, it is *nutritious*.

Therefore, the qualities of Earth are *heavy, dense, solid, cold, static, drying,* and *nutritious*. (See TABLE 5.1, The Attributes of The Five Phases)

Without the Earth Phase, our bodies would not have cellular structures or bones.

TABLE–5-1

THE ATTRIBUTES OF THE FIVE PHASES

SPACE	AIR	FIRE	WATER	EARTH
Rarefied	Movement	Hot	Wet	Heavy
Cold	Cold	Fluid	Cold	Dense
Movement	Dry	Sharp	Heavy	Solid
Light	Rough	Light	Slow	Cold
Clear	Light	Clear	Dull	Static
Subtle	Clear	Drying	Fluid	Drying
Expansive	Subtle	Spreading		Nutritious

The Five Phases of Chinese Medicine

The Five Phases of Chinese Medicine are slightly different in terminology from Ayurveda but the concepts are the same. Like Native American medicine, The Five Phases of Chinese Medicine are depicted as a wheel with one Phase in the center.

The Phases of Fire, Water, and Earth are essentially the same; Wood and Metal are different terminologies that can be somewhat correlated to the original Five Phases of Ayurveda although it is not exact.

Wood

The Wood Phase in Chinese Medicine is expansive and is associated with the attribute of wind and movement and the Liver and Gallbladder Systems.

The expansive (more Space Phase) and movement (more Air Phase) are also attributes of the Space Phase. Therefore, the Chinese Medicine Wood Phase appears to correlate with the Space Phase.

Notes

Metal

The Metal Phase in Chinese Medicine is associated with dryness and contraction (a quality of cold) and the Lung and Large Intestine Systems. While dryness (more Air Phase), and coldness (more Space Phase) are also associated with the Space Phase, the Lung and Large Intestine Systems are correlated with the Air Phase.

Table–5-2

CORRELATED PHASES

AYURVEDA	CHINESE MEDICINE
Space	Wood
Air	Metal
Fire	Fire
Water	Water
Earth	Earth (center)

In the next chapter, we will see how The Five Phases are combined in different ways by Nature to impart our ability to experience life especially how it relates to herbal medicine and food.

Notes

Chapter 6:

Into Perception: The Six Tastes

The universe does not seem to exist without a perceiver of that universe.

—Fred Alan Wolf, physicist[1]

The Six Tastes are made up of different combinations of The Five Phases. The Five Phase combinations impart the therapeutic properties of herbs (and foods) that allow us to use herbal medicine more effectively and safely.

Taste stimulates our nervous system by the chemical reactions that begin with our tongue. When we say an herb has a heating Taste, it means the *effect* of that herb is heating. It does not mean the herb actually imparts heat to the body.

From a scientific point of view, our nervous systems contain sensory neurons, called nociceptors, that respond to different types of stimuli by sending nerve signals to the spinal cord and/or brain. Different types of stimulation of a nociceptor will lead to different responses such as the sensation of heat.[2]

Ayurveda has classified Six Tastes while Chinese Medicine addresses Five Tastes. Both modalities have interesting and enlightening differences and similarities that will be discussed in this chapter.

The Six Tastes of Ayurveda

The detailed information about The Six Tastes comes to us from Ayurveda. The properties of The Six Tastes transmit the actions of The Five Phases into the body that are necessary to maintain health. It is why Ayurveda advocates eating all six Tastes at every meal.

The Five Phases when combined differently convey The Six Tastes—Sweet, Sour, Salty, Pungent, Bitter, and Astringent. In other words, when combining The Five Phases in six

Notes

different combinations, the result is the transmission of the attributes of The Five Phases that stimulate the nervous system producing the experience of The Six Tastes.

The ancients did not have direct knowledge of nociceptors or the molecules that produce the Tastes, but they had acute insight from experience into the reactions that the Tastes produced. For example, knowledge of the chemical makeup of cayenne pepper is not necessary to know that it conveys a sense of heat to the taste buds, can burn and dry your mouth, and create inflammation or a sensation of heat.

If one can accurately *taste* (a chemical reaction) an herb, one can know how to use it and apply it effectively. Taste is, most likely, the way ancient herbal medicines were discovered and used. Taste and smell are probably how our animals know what herbs to eat when their bodies need some help.

The ancients also noticed that certain Tastes have an affinity for certain organ-systems. See Table-6-1.

Table–6-1

THE SIX TASTES & ORGAN-SYSTEMS

TASTE	ORGAN-SYSTEM
Sweet	Metabolic
Sour	Liver
Salty	Kidney
Pungent	Lung
Bitter	Heart
Astringent	Colon

The Sweet Taste

The Sweet Taste and its qualities are generated from the combination of the Phases of Earth and Water.

- Combining Earth and Water produces soil that has the water and *nutrients* present to promote growth and build cellular structure.
- Earth and Water together also can make mud, depending on the proportion of water to soil, that has a *smooth* and soothing quality.
- Mud is also *heavy, slow* and *damp*—qualities of the Earth and Water Phases.
- We know from experience that eating a lot of sweet foods *promotes growth* or makes you gain weight.
- Sweet foods also make you feel *heavy* and feeling heavier would make you move *slowly*, feel dull with increased mucus or *damp*.

Notes

We call Sweet foods comfort foods because of their soothing and smoothing qualities. The Sweet Taste is also necessary as it provides nourishment for our bodies, in the form of *nutrients* from the Earth Phase, to maintain our bodily structures, such as bones and cellular structures. Sweet is also *cooling* which is why we prefer to eat more fruit in the summertime.

Foods that are considered Sweet do not actually need to have the sugary sweet taste. Animal based products are especially sweet due to their excessive protein and high caloric content (Earth Phase). (See Chapter 15.)

Table–6-2

THE SWEET TASTE:
Attributes of Earth & Water

EARTH	WATER
Heavy	Wet
Dense	Cold
Solid	Heavy
Cold	Slow
Static	Dull
Nutritious	Fluid

Table–6-3

EXAMPLES OF THE SWEET TASTE:
Combined Phases of Earth & Water

FOODS	HERBS
Grains	Slippery Elm
Wheat	Marshmallow Root
Nuts	Psyllium
Fruit	Comfrey
Animal products	Aloe Vera

The Sour Taste

Notes

The Phases that make-up the Sour Taste are Earth and Fire.

- From the Earth and Fire Phases is derived the qualities of *heat* and *dryness.*
- From the Earth Phase, we get the *nutrient* quality that gives us growth and the cold quality to moderate the *heat* from the Fire Phase.

Combining the Earth and Fire Phases we have an improvement in metabolism and digestive ability since these functions are dependent on the chemical *heat* of transformation.

With increased metabolism comes an increase in energy supported by the *nutrient* quality of the Earth Phase.

In addition, the Fire and Earth Phases impart a *drying* action that can eliminate mucus or damp quality in the body.

Consuming too much of the Sour Taste can result in a dry mouth, thirst, and weight gain.

Table–6-4

THE SOUR TASTE:
Attributes of Fire & Earth

FIRE	EARTH
Hot	Heavy
Fluid	Dense
Sharp	Solid
Light	Cold
Clear	Static
Drying	Nutritious

Table–6-5

EXAMPLES OF THE SOUR TASTE:
Combined Phases of Earth & Fire

FOODS	HERBS
Lemon	Rosehips
Orange Peel	Hawthorne Berry
Vinegar	Raspberry
Beets	Schisandra
Blackberry	

Notes

The Salty Taste

The Phases that make-up the Salty Taste are Fire and Water. An acid, which is heating, is created when inert salt compounds are dissolved in water.

- Combining the attributes of Fire and Water conveys *moisture*, its softening effects come from the Water Phase, and *heat* from the Fire Phase that helps digestion.
- Consuming too much of the Salty Taste would have a laxative effect and make you feel thirsty and *dry*.

Large amounts of the Salty Taste would cause nausea or vomiting, skin to wrinkle, burning sensations, and the teeth to loosen or fall out.

Table–6-6

THE SALTY TASTE:
Attributes of Fire & Water

FIRE	WATER
Hot	Wet
Fluid	Cold
Sharp	Heavy
Light	Slow
Clear	Dull
Drying	Fluid

Table–6-7

EXAMPLES OF THE SALTY TASTE:
Combined Phases of Water & Fire

FOODS	HERBS
Seaweeds	Seaweeds
Sea Salt	Epsom Salts
Epsom Salts	Parsley Root
Celery	Seashells
Parsley Root	

The Pungent Taste

The Pungent Taste is made up of the Phases of Fire and Air.

- The Fire Phase conveys the quality of *heat* improving digestion and having a *drying* effect.
- The Phase of Air brings the qualities of wind, *movement* and *lightness.*

Combined, the quality of *wind* or *movement* supports the quality of *heat* by fanning or increasing the fire. Therefore, the *heat* in the Pungent Taste improves digestion, burns up mucus and dampness.

The *wind* and *movement* will also break up obstructions and masses and generally clear the system.

Too much of the Pungent Taste can cause burning sensations, thirst from heat and dryness, depletion from consumption (transformation) of tissues, and dizziness from uprising heat.

Table–6-8

THE PUNGENT TASTE:
Attributes of Air & Fire

FIRE	AIR
Hot	Movement
Fluid	Cold
Sharp	Dry
Light	Rough
Clear	Light
Drying	Clear
	Subtle

Notes

Notes

Table–6-9

EXAMPLES OF THE PUNGENT TASTE: *Combined Phases of Air & Fire*

FOODS	HERBS
Onion	Basil
Garlic	Ginger
Chilies	Black Pepper
Mustard	Cloves
Radish	Nutmeg
Watercress	Cinnamon
Leeks	Oregano
	Rosemary
	Sage
	Thyme

The Bitter Taste

The Bitter Taste consists of the Phases of Air and Space.

- Air and Space Phases have the attributes of *coldness, movement*, and *lightness.* Therefore, the Bitter Taste has a significant cooling and moving effects as well as an ability to alleviate heaviness.
- The *cooling* effect gives the Bitter Taste detoxifying properties by reducing heat (infection, inflammation) and the ability to reduce fevers.
- The *movement* quality helps digestion by moving food through the system keeping it from stagnating and accumulating. It also has a dispersing or detoxifying effect.

If too much of the Bitter Taste were to be consumed, which is rare since most diets lack this Taste, one might experience emaciation, weakness, rough and dry skin, and dizziness.

Notes

Table–6-10

THE BITTER TASTE:
Attributes of Space & Air

FIRE	WATER
Movement	Rarefied
Cold	Cold
Dry	Movement
Rough	Light
Light	Clear
Clear	Subtle
Subtle	

Table–6-11

EXAMPLES OF THE BITTER TASTE:
Combined Phases of Air & Space

FOODS	HERBS
Coffee	Dandelion
Cocoa	Echinacea
Olives	Goldenseal
Citrus Peel	Oregon Grape Root
Chicory	Barberry
Escarole	Aloe
Hops	Gentian
Quinine	Chocolate

Notes

The Astringent Taste

The Astringent Taste consists of the Phases of Air and Earth.

- Air and Earth Phases have *drying* properties as Air will dry and Earth will dry by absorbing moisture.

Therefore, the Astringent Taste can alleviate excessive secretions such as diarrhea, bleeding, and sweating, tighten and constrict tissues and raise prolapsed organs.

Too much of the Astringent Taste can be drying causing dry skin and premature aging, constipation, thirst, and heart pain.

Table–6-12

THE ASTRINGENT TASTE:
Attributes of Air & Earth

AIR	EARTH
Movement	Heavy
Cold	Dense
Dry	Solid
Rough	Cold
Light	Static
Clear	Nutritious
Subtle	

Table–6-13

EXAMPLES OF THE ASTRINGENT TASTE:
Combined Phases of Air & Earth

FOODS	HERBS
Unripe banana	White Oak Bark
Pomegranate	Witch Hazel
Chickpeas	Plantain
Raspberries	Lotus Seed
Black Tea	Mullein
	Uva Ursi

The Five Tastes of Chinese Medicine

Notes

Chinese Medicine addresses Five Tastes. Some of Chinese Medicine's Five Tastes are the same and some are slightly different in the proportions and combinations of the Phases. These additional Tastes have been incorporated as they provide more terms to qualify our experiences.

The Phases of Sweet, Salty, and Sour remain the same. The Bitter Taste is slightly altered. The additional Tastes are Aromatic, Acrid, and Bland.

According to Chinese Medicine, "Acrid substances disperse and move; sweet substances tonify, . . . bitter substances drain and dry; sour substances are astringent and prevent or reverse the abnormal leakage of fluids and energy . . . salty substances purge and soften; bland substances leech out dampness and promote urination."[3]

The Aromatic Taste

According to Bensky and Gamble's *Materia Medica,* Aromatic is not a Taste but a temperature characteristic that has more of the Fire Phase. The Phases of the Aromatic "Taste" are Fire, Air, and Space that are similar to Pungent except more warming and dispersing with the "ability to penetrate . . . and revive a particular function. . . "[4] The penetrating action is an attribute of Fire and Air Phases. Therefore, refer to Pungent for details about this Taste.

The Acrid Taste in Chinese Medicine

The definition in Western dictionaries refers to acrid and pungent as the same or similar.

However, in *A Barefoot Doctor's Manual,* acrid has a peppery taste,[5] and according to Bensky and Gamble's *Materia Medica,* "Acrid substances disperse and move. . . "[6] The only Phases that have the attributes of dispersion and movement are Space and Air. This is like Bitter but with the Space Phase predominant giving Acrid its increased dispersing quality.

Most of the herbs labeled as Acrid in the *Materia Medica* are cooling or cold in Energy, though some have the added Phase of Fire giving it a more penetrating quality. The *Materia Medica* states that Acrid can be divided into cool and warm. ". . . an acrid, warm substance can be used for externally-contracted cold; an acrid, cool substance for externally-contracted heat, . . . "[7]

Therefore, the Phases of the Acrid Taste are Space and Air with the occasional addition of Fire.

Notes

TABLE–6-14

THE ACRID TASTE:
Attributes of Space & Air

SPACE	AIR
Rarefied	Movement
Cold	Cold
Movement	Dry
Light	Rough
Clear	Light
Subtle	Clear
	Subtle

The properties of the Acrid Taste are the same as Bitter in Ayurveda. However, in Chinese Medicine "bitter substances drain and dry"[8] and therefore the Bitter Taste in Chinese Medicine may have some of the Earth Phase giving it additional drying and draining properties.

The Bland Taste in Chinese Medicine

The Bland Taste in Chinese Medicine consists of Earth and Air. This is like Astringent except the Earth Phase is more predominant. The larger proportion of the Earth Phase, that absorbs water, is drying. The heaviness of the Earth Phase also moves water downward and the Air Phase helps move water out of the body.

According to Bensky and Gamble's *Materia Medica,* Bland herbs "leach out dampness and promote urination."[9] That is, these herbs act as diuretics.

Notes

Table–6-15

THE BLAND TASTE IN CHINESE MEDICINE:
Attributes of Earth & Air

EARTH	AIR
Heavy	Movement
Dense	Cold
Solid	Dry
Cold	Rough
Static	Light
Nutritious	Clear
	Subtle

Table–6-16

EXAMPLES OF BLAND TASTE IN CHINESE MEDICINE:
Combined Phases of Earth & Air

WESTERN HERBS	EASTERN HERBS
Lysimachia	Poria *(fu ling)*
Red Clover Flower	Polypori *(zhu ling)*
	Coicis *(yi yi ren)*

Notes

Chapter 7:

The Big Bang Theory: Ayurveda

It is becoming ever more apparent that mysticism, or the perennial [Eastern] philosophy, as it is sometimes called, provides the most consistent philosophical background to the new scientific paradigm.

—Fritjof Capra, physicist[1]

Ayurveda is the earliest form of medicine on our planet originating in India well over 5,000 years ago. It was, at first, a Vedic oral tradition before it was eventually written down. From northern India, the knowledge and wisdom of Ayurveda spread and was modified as it expanded throughout the world. Ayurveda is The Big Bang of medicine.

Cosmologists believe that our universe came into being about 13.8 billion years ago from a tiny, dense state to a sudden expansion called The Big Bang Theory. Technically the Big Bang Theory does not describe an explosive origin of the universe, but how it has continued to evolve in an expansive motion. It is the beginning of our time and space.[2]

According to astronomers, the universe is still expanding as evidenced by our ability to measure the light, called redshift, received from distant galaxies. Some physicists believe that our universe will continue to expand, and some believe that at some point it will begin to contract and then expand again. Physicists are unable to confirm or disprove any of these theories yet.

This constant expansion and contraction, as if the cosmos were alive with the breath of life known as *prana*, is very similar to Hindu mysticism on which Ayurveda is based. Modern physics is now proving the validity of some of the mystical theories of Eastern philosophy on the nature of the universe. From Fritjof Capra:

> *The world view of the Eastern mystics shares with the bootstrap philosophy of modern physics not only an emphasis on the mutual interrelation and self-consistency of all phenomena, but also the denial of fundamental constituents of matter.*[3]

The Philosophy of Ayurveda

Notes

According to Ayurveda, before the beginning, or what science calls The Big Bang there was Awareness of Oneness. Within the original Awareness of Oneness, arose a desire to experience itself that created Duality of Awareness or Experience. This Duality-Awareness of Experience created the energy of friction and the manifestation of Energy or *Prana*. Some of this manifested Energy condensed becoming matter. To understand matter, one needs to experience it, and so this trinity, Awareness, Experience, and Energy/Matter came into being, with the result, our physical universe with its diverse attributes. Physicist Amit Goswami explains, "Without the immanent world of manifestation, there would be no soul, no self that experiences itself as separate from the objects it perceives."[4]

While the above is a mystical interpretation of the beginnings of our universe, physicist Fritjof Capra agrees that the mystical and spiritual perspective has validity.

> *The new worldview is an ecological worldview that is grounded, ultimately, in spiritual awareness. Therefore, it is not surprising that the new paradigm, as it emerges in physics and in the other sciences, will be in harmony with many ideas in spiritual traditions.*[5]

Ayurveda also discusses the Theory of Relativity in its concept of *maya*. *Maya* is the illusion of assuming the forms, or matter of the world, is reality instead of knowing they are the desire of the mind (free-will) to measure and define. In other words, if your point of view is mechanistic, you are under the illusion of matter, deluded. If your point of view is one of relativity—knowing that everything is a dynamic oneness of energy—then you come to see the world as it really is.[6]

> *The inconsistency of the modern mechanist is: If this were merely a material universe and man only a machine, such a man would be wholly unable to recognize himself as such a machine, and likewise would such a machine-man be wholly unconscious of the fact of the existence of such a material universe.*[7]

It is difficult to see beyond the time-space realm when one is limited by a mind conceived in time and space since, "Time-space minds, organized out of the energies of time and space, are subject to the mechanisms of time and space."[8] Therefore, our ability to perceive the nature of the universe is limited to the realm of the mechanistic mind. It is why the Eastern mystics' "models of reality constitute a more appropriate philosophical background to modern physics than the models of Western philosophy."[9]

Through theories of relativity and quantum physics, modern physics discovered that in observing energy/matter, awareness, as the observer, influences matter being perceived.[10] Therefore, modern physics has brought us full circle to what the ancients knew to be accurate reality. Modern physics has brought together the science of physics and the poetry of life—matter and experience are one. Awareness can manipulate energy-matter since it is originally Awareness that created it.

Notes

The universe is neither mechanical nor magical; it is a creation of mind and a mechanism of law. But while in practical application the laws of nature operate in what seems to be the dual realms of the physical and the spiritual, in reality they are one.[11]

Ayurveda for over 5,000 years has continually valued what modern physics has shown to be reality—the foundation of life is consciousness and body or energy-matter, but the essence of life is the spirit-awareness, the "heart of matter"—part of the living cosmic web of life. Our lives are physics and poetry, matter and expression, context and awareness. It is this fundamental understanding and wisdom of all aspects of life that renders Ayurveda so valuable in maintaining our health.

The Fundamentals of Ayurveda

Ayurveda is a vital science and art-healing system that provides guidance for living in harmony with our inner, microcosmic, and outer, macrocosmic, environments as well as other beings around us. It's way of teaching us is very poetic, because life is poetic, with much more going on between the lines and the wave-particles of potential matter than is readily apparent by just the energy-material "facts" of the wave-particles themselves. This is said with the understanding that our minds manufacture fact. ". . . we develop the fact by giving it further order, form and structure."[12]

Ayurveda is unique in that it clearly informs us how to live in harmony with Nature. It is the "wisdom of living." One may call it the original ecological worldview where the fundamental interdependence of all living systems is primary. Ayurveda encompasses all aspects of life—our physical bodies, our thoughts and emotions, our spiritual connections, our relationships and inter-relationships to each other and the other living systems in our environment. Ayurveda teaches us how to maintain a dynamic harmony with these concepts to maintain and regain our health.

Ayurveda has many aspects to it covering diverse topics such as: yoga, meditation, surgery (plastic surgery techniques that are still used today), acupuncture, psychology, rejuvenation, herbal medicine, and much more. Many of Ayurveda's disciplines are still practiced today.

Ayurveda in the Clinic

In Eastern medicine diagnosing a condition is not a simple matter of naming a disease. A Western diagnosis does not give the Eastern medicine practitioner enough information. The same disease can manifest differently in different people (context) which is why the same treatment does not always work with everybody.

For example, diagnosing a disorder in Ayurveda is very complex. The examination includes an assessment of the pulses (See Chapter 10), urine, stool, tongue, eyes, skin, speech and voice, and general appearance. Additional examinations are made to assess digestive capacity, personal habits, body appearance, and the person's resilience. Also considered, is the most recent reason for the illness, symptoms, various diagnostic tests, and pathogenesis.[13]

Notes

Since the expression of genes is dependent on one's environment, Ayurveda emphasizes the importance of environmental factors on health, such as daily routine, seasonal changes, and lifestyle factors such as diet, regular exercise, and appropriate herbal tonics.

After having discussed the Phases, Tastes, and The Functional Principles, you may begin to appreciate that there could be Hot, Cold, Damp, Dry conditions or any combinations thereof in assessing a disorder in Eastern Medicine. It can be a challenging task and one that takes many years of clinical experience.

Ayurveda and Herbal Medicine

As Ayurveda relates to herbal medicine—"Man as microcosm contains within himself all the elemental, mineral, vegetable and animal kingdoms."[14] On the macrocosmic level, all life is nurtured by cosmic energy or light, that plants capture. Plants then nurture us with this cosmic-light energy on the physical, psychological, and spiritual levels. The physicist Fritjof Capra says, ". . . green plants link the earth and the sky."[15]

"Plants exist to transmute light into life and . . . The human being transmutes life into consciousness through perception."[16] Perception is the act of observation or experience. Each plant, herb or food, has its own special wavelengths of light-energy (as demonstrated in gas chromatography) or consciousness. When the plant is digested it will bring balanced function to that part of the body akin to those wavelengths. This is how herbs or foods are known to work on certain parts of the body.

Ahamkara—Personality

Ahamkara, or Personality, is the manifestation of the original Awareness to experience itself as the Duality of Awareness. It is the personality that comes from, but is different from, the Awareness of Oneness. Personality is what makes you an individual, a unique identity, your personal awareness and perspective.

The personality form is the *pattern* aspect of a living being; it connotes the *arrangement* of energies, and this, plus life and motion, is the *mechanism* of creature existence.[17] The "arrangement of energies" are the combination of The Five Phases that make up the *doshas* described later in this chapter; "life" is the vital spark or *prana* that enlivens the body; "motion" is the process of activity involved in the ongoing expression of the system's pattern of organization.

The Three Gunas—Qualities

From the Duality of Awareness and our personality come the three basic *gunas* or qualities of our individual expression. All physical creation is made up of the three basic *gunas* or qualities of expression, a process from which The Five Phases spring. From *Sattva* arises Space; from *Rajas* comes Fire; and from *Tamas* results Earth. Between Space and Fire there is Air, and between Fire and Earth there is Water. (See Chapter 5.)

Notes

Sattva, contains the subjective world, your personal and unique awareness and perspective, your personality. It is the principle of free-will, potential energy, intelligence and harmony. *Sattva*-Perception encompasses the higher values and qualities of truth, beauty, goodness, honesty, humility, and compassion. It is awareness that knows the "heart of matter" but is different from matter; it exists in the spaces between matter. *Sattva* is the personality-free-will concept that can choose to be the observer.

In terms of modern physics *Sattva*-Perception is the awareness that can make the choice, out of all the wave-particle-like patterns of probabilities that exist, which probability is to be perceived. By making that free-will choice to become the perceiver, *Sattva*-Perception has chosen which probability of reality the former perceiver, and now participator, will focus. At that instant *Sattva* becomes *Rajas*-participator. Before that decision, *Sattva*-Perception is simply an undifferentiated choice-concept, or free-will, that remains a part of, but different from, the Awareness of Oneness. In the words of Fritjof Capra,

> *They [Eastern mystics] go much further, and in deep meditation they arrive at a point where the distinction between observer and observed breaks down completely, where subject and object fuse into unified undifferentiated whole.*[18]

Rajas, is the Participator, the active part of the seemingly objective world, the mind, the vital life force or energy of movement, the principle of kinetic energy, activity, emotion, as well as turbulence and discordance. *Rajas*-Participator encompasses the psychologically dynamic qualities of power, prestige, authority, and control. *Rajas* is the act of observation. Fritjof Capra explains the role of the observer in science, "... the scientist cannot play the role of a detached objective observer, but becomes involved in the world he observes to the extent that he influences the properties of the observed objects."[19]

It is *Rajas*-Participator that in the act of perceiving becomes involved in the world he observes and thereby affects the world he observes. Therefore, the objects perceived by *Rajas* are brought forth through the action of perception. *Rajas* is the Duality of Awareness or Experience.

Modern physicist John Wheeler describes it thus,

> *Nothing is more important about the quantum principle than this, that it destroys the concept of the world as "sitting out there," with the observer safely separated from it... To describe what has happened, one has to cross out that old word "observer," and put in its place the new word "participator." In some strange sense the universe is a participatory universe.*[20]

Tamas, the Perceived, contains the objective or material world. *Tamas*-Perceived is the principle of inertia, darkness, dullness, and resistance. *Tamas* encompasses the psychological qualities of fear, lassitude, ignorance, and hedonism. *Tamas* is the observed.

In modern physics *Tamas*-Perceived are the atoms and their particles, the matter itself. The Duality of Awareness or Rajas-Participator creates, due to duality, the energy of friction that then manifests as Energy and then condenses to become matter. *Tamas*-Perceived has no meaning/value unless *Rajas* perceives it and *Sattva*-Perception chooses to perceive it and give it value. Capra confirms these concepts in the following:

The crucial feature of atomic physics is that the human observer is not only necessary to observe the properties of an object, but is necessary even to define these properties. In atomic physics, we cannot talk about the properties of an object as such. They are only meaningful in the context to the object's interaction with the observer.[21]

Notes

Therefore, we have the concepts of awareness of Perception, the one who determines value; Participator or one who takes the action to get involved in the drama of perception; and the inert object to be Perceived. The object is fact and is measurable. Action or energy can also be measured by mass and speed. But awareness, the context, cannot be measured but it gives value/meaning to the action and the object, the "heart" creating and then perceiving the "matter." Awareness is indeed the "heart of matter."

The systems theory of cognition developed by Humberto Maturana and Francisco Varela in 1978, also called the Santiago theory, states the Ayurvedic concepts of Sattva, Rajas, Tamas as follows according to Capra:

The new concept of cognition, the process of knowing, is thus much broader than that of thinking. It involves perception [Sattva], emotion [Tamas], and action [Rajas]—the entire process of life.[22]

Understanding the three qualities, Perception, Perceiver, Perceived, provides insight into, not only the reality of the interdependence our existence, but the psychological makeup of someone who predominantly possesses those qualities.

Dosha

The new form of insight can perhaps best be called Undivided Wholeness in Flowing Movement.

—David Bohm, physicist[23]

The term *dosha* translates as fault or mistake. Functionally, *dosha* is the by-products of the process of cellular metabolism, from the air, food, and drink we ingest. It includes everything from heat to the waste products our bodies manufacture.

When the *doshas* are balanced and *moving out of the system,* health [self-organization] is maintained. If one or more of the *doshas* accumulate in the body, disharmony results and eventually disease. That is, the by-products of cellular metabolism, the waste products, must not be allowed to accumulate in the body or ill health will result. It is described by Dr. Larry Dossey as a "biodance" of chemicals entering and exiting the body that accounts for its rhythmic regeneration and, therefore, health.

According to systems theory, developed in the 1940s by biologist Ludwig von Bertalanffy (1901-1972), living systems function with a "flowing balance."[24] That is, in living systems the structure is relatively stable but within it there is a constant flow of matter. Stagnation in the body, therefore, is contrary to Nature and produces illness. As

Notes

Capra states, "A constant flow of energy and matter through the system is necessary for self-organization to take place."[25]

This concept can be illustrated by a wood stove and flue. The fire in the stove will heat a room if the ash (waste product) is removed from the stove and flue regularly. If the ash is not consistently removed there could be one of several outcomes—the fuel will not burn properly and the fire will go out resulting in a cold room, or the fire will continue to burn but smoke will fill the room that will cause you to leave the heated room. Either scenario results in your being uncomfortable.

The structure of the stove remains the same but the constant burning of wood in the stove is being transformed to create heat. The waste product from the transformation of wood into heat, is the ash that must be removed to keep the system functioning properly. In a living system, the heat would be utilized for other metabolic processes, also producing waste products that must be removed, to keep the system healthy.

In Ayurveda, there is a working interrelationship between the tissues of the nervous system and the dosha of Vata; the digestive system and the dosha of Pitta; and the quantity and quality of body fluids and the dosha of Kapha. By observing the condition of these tissues and their interdependent functions, disorders in the system can be determined.

Table–7-1

THE DOSHAS & TISSUES

DOSHA	TISSUE
Vata	Nervous System
Pitta	Bile, Enzymes
Kapha	Bones, Body Fluids

In Ayurveda, excess Vata will manifest as nervousness and anxiety; excess Pitta will manifest as irritability and anger; and excess Kapha will manifest as sluggishness and depression.

Table–7-2

THE DOSHAS & EMOTIONS

DOSHA	EMOTION
Vata	Nervousness
Pitta	Irritability
Kapha	Sluggishness, depression

Notes

In Ayurveda, Vata will be provoked by changes in the weather and seasons, such as Spring and Fall, as well as excess wind, dryness, and cold; Pitta will be provoked by hot and humid weather and summertime; and Kapha will be provoked by cold and wet weather and wintertime.

Table–7-3

THE DOSHAS & ENVIRONMENT

DOSHA	EMOTION
Vata	Fall, Spring—wind, dry, cold
Pitta	Summer—hot, humid
Kapha	Winter—cold, wet

Prakruti versus Vikruti
or Flowing Balance versus Disease

Every living entity on the planet has all three *doshas* inherent in its makeup or it could not exist. What differs from person to person is the *proportion* of the doshas. An individual's unique *doshic* balance is determined at conception and is called *Prakruti* or "original constitution." It is the unique original constitution we are constantly trying to maintain to retain our health.

The out of balance state of disorder or disease is called *Vikruti* or "unbalanced state." If you are out of balance you would be treated according to your unbalanced state to eliminate the accumulation/stagnation of one or more of the *doshas*. For example, in your unbalanced state you may be given a food-guideline different from your original constitution to help bring your system back into balance.

The Three Doshas—Constitutions

Having discussed The Five Phases in detail in Chapter 5, we can expound on how they transfer their qualities to our bodies to make up the three basic constitutional tendencies or *doshas* of Ayurveda.

The three *doshas* or constitutions—Vata, Pitta, Kapha—are created from The Five Phases. Each constitution is a combination of mainly two of The Five Phases, one of which predominates—Vata is the principle of Air; Pitta is the principle of Fire; Kapha is the principle of Water. Every constitution has its physical (Perceived), mental-emotional (Perceiver), and spiritual (Perception) tendencies due to the relationship of combinations and proportions of The Five Phases present.

In other words, the tendencies of expression of the constitution are determined by the interrelationships of The Five Phases. This is like quantum physics where a subatomic wave-particle has a probability to occur (express) depending on its interrelationships between various complex processes, which, in this case are The Five Phases. These in turn, can only be understood by the interactions with other relationships as discussed next.

Notes

Vata
Air & Space Phases
Perception
The Principle of Air

Vata
Mind a windswept landscape
Slight for resistance
No friction for fire.

Lithe as whip
Moves at the touch of a thought
For its own sake.

Agitated leaves in the breeze
Jumpy is joy
Slumber obscure.

Fickle is the day
Random desire
Merging rations fitful.

Arid topical zone
Irregular grit
Forgetful thirst.

Clear for inspiration
Artist in flight
No landings here.
—J. Shamosh

Vata is mainly the Air Phase with Space as the secondary Phase. The Vata dosha can be equated with the functions of the central nervous system.

- Vata *dosha* can be demonstrated by a *cool windy* day.
- On such a day, everything is *moving* in an *erratic* manner. One minute the wind may be blowing vigorously and the next it may stop altogether.
- The wind makes you feel cool or *cold* that can irritate your nervous system, the never-sleeping, constantly active part of our systems.
- Your skin may become *dry* and, over several days of this experience, your skin may feel *rough* (chapped) so you will feel the need to moisturize it.
- The leaves of the trees and plants *move*, tremble and flutter.
- The wind may pick up soil and erode the landscape making its surface *rough*.

Table–7-4

VATA: PERCEPTION

AIR	SPACE
Movement	Rarefied
Cold	Cold
Dry	Movement
Rough	Light
Light	Clear
Clear	Subtle
Subtle	Expansive

Notes

While you cannot see the wind because it is *clear* and *subtle* you know its effects by the experiences and observations mentioned above.

Vata is the *subtle* energy governing *movement*. It is the motivating force for all the other Phases. For example, it is the wind of Vata that picks up and moves earth.

When Vata *dosha* is in balance, it regulates all flowing movement in the body. As such, it is the constantly active *nervous system* that manifests Vata imbalances. Therefore, all the functions controlled by the nervous system, are regulated by Vata such as: the beating of your heart, breathing, eating and intestinal movements, urination, bowel elimination, movement of limbs and eyes, sensory acuity, and sleeping. Anything in the body that moves is Vata in expression.

In modern physics Vata can be equated with the "fundamental 'restlessness' of matter. . . "[26] that defies confinement. . . . the being of matter [that] cannot be separated from its activity."[27]

Table–7-5

TENDENCIES OF VATA DOSHA[28]

Dry skin, hair, lips, tongue, throat; constipation
Slight muscles, bones, thin body frame; light sleep; underweight
Cold hands, feet; poor circulation; avoids cold, loves heat; muscle stiffness
Rough, cracked skin, nails, hair; cracking joints
Subtle fear, anxiety, insecurity; small muscle twitches or tremors
Fast walking, talking, thinking; multitasking, scattered thoughts and mind, restless; mood swings
Easily understands and forgets; clairvoyant, perceptive; clear mind, creative; tends to loneliness
Dark complexion, hair, eyes; brown spots, moles

Notes

Pitta
Fire & Water Phases
Perceiver
The Principle of Fire

Pitta
Radiant heat
Furious fire when stirred
Touch warm
Surface like Mars

Piercing psyche
Imaginative insight
Decisive determination
Winsome wit

Data digested
Feasts transformed
Words a banquet
Intelligence feeding

Deeds doing
Feats finished
Poise plenty
Confidence certain.
—J. Shamosh

Table–7-6

PITTA: PERCEIVER

FIRE	WATER
Hot	Wet
Fluid	Cold
Sharp	Heavy
Light	Slow
Clear	Dull
Drying	Fluid
Spreading	

Pitta is mainly Fire with Water as the secondary Phase. Therefore, Pitta is the quality of heat. The corresponding Water Phase is the moderating effect on the Fire Phase and also provides moisture. (See the Fire Phase, Chapter 5.) The Pitta dosha can be equated with the metabolic processes of the body.

Fire provides heat and radiance and has an upward movement that can affect the upper parts of the body.

Heat transforms and dries substances and has a penetrating quality due to the excitation of atoms transmitted from one substance to another. It is the basis of digestion known in Ayurveda as *agni.* Anything having the property of heat is Pitta.

Pitta determines digestion and digestive secretions, such as bile and enzymes, chemical reactions, bodily heat, hunger, skin luster, and visual acuity. Therefore, in balance, Pitta has excellent digestion and appetite, good metabolism, warm, soft and lustrous skin, and good vision.

Pitta is ruled by the First Law of Thermodynamics stating that heat must be supplied for an engine to produce work. In this case Pitta is the engine (the doer, achiever, perceiver) and the heat is supplied by the thermochemical reactions of metabolism, which in Pitta, is usually excellent.

Notes

Table–7-7

TENDENCIES OF PITTA DOSHA[29]

Good digestion, appetite; warm temperature; avoids heat
Sharp, distinct features; good absorption/digestion; sharp mind memory and comprehension; tends to irritability
Light to medium frame; photophobic; fair to reddish skin; bright eyes
Loose stools; excess sweat, thirst, urine
Spreading rashes, acne, inflammation
Soft, oily skin, hair
Red, flushed skin, eyes, cheeks, nose
Yellow eyes, skin, urine; heartburn, bitter taste, easily angered

Notes

Kapha
Water & Earth Phases
Perceived
The Principle of Water

Kapha
Balmy is the heart
Cool is the essence
Heavy in mass
Buoyant of spirit.

Measured movement
Leisured days
Load increasing
Burdensome body.

Mighty muscle
Enduring endurance
Mindful memory
Dampness diminishes.

Fondness for forgiving
Contented devotion
Faithful friend
Patient partner.

Gentle giving
Deep desire
Consistent caring
Loving lives.
—J. Shamosh

Table–7-8

KAPHA: PERCEIVED

WATER	EARTH
Wet	Heavy
Cold	Dense
Heavy	Solid
Slow	Cold
Dull	Static
Fluid	Nutritious
	Drying

Notes

The Kapha *dosha* is a combination of the Water and Earth Phases with Water being primary. The Kapha *dosha* can be equated with the lymphatic system, immune system, adipose tissue, mucus and mucoid systems, and bones.

Because of the Water and Earth Phases, Kapha *dosha* tends to be cold, damp, heavy, firm, stable, lubricating, and responsible for bodily growth.

In balance, Kapha exhibits strength and stamina, firmness, good immunity, stability, regularity, lubrication of joints, regular appetite, slow digestion, sound sleep.

Kapha is ruled by Isaac Newton's First Law of Motion of inertia stating that an object either remains at rest or continues to move at a constant velocity unless acted upon by an external force. The resistance to acceleration is due to Kapha's generally larger mass and gravity's pull on that mass.

Table–7-9

TENDENCIES OF KAPHA DOSHA[30]

Heavy bones, muscles; large frame; tends to overweight; grounded
Slow walker, talker; slow digestion, metabolism; slow reactions
Cool clammy skin; steady appetite, thirst; colds, congestion, coughs
Oily skin, hair
Excess salivation; congestion in chest, sinuses, throat, head
Smooth skin; gentle mind; calm nature
Dense padding of fat; thick skin, hair, nails; plump, firm and solid muscles
Soft pleasing look; loving, caring, compassion, kindness, forgiveness
Loves sitting, sleeping, doing nothing
Loves to hug; deeply attached in love and relationships, possessive
Obstructions and accumulations lead to obesity
Pale complexion; white mucus, tongue coating

How Your *Doshas* Are Determined

Your *doshas* are determined ultimately by pulse diagnosis—both original constitution and unbalanced state. Pulse diagnosis will give the exact proportions of Vata, Pitta, and Kapha both in balance and out of balance (See Chapter 10).

Your *doshas* can also be determined by careful and trained observation. However, for your information you can use Tables 7-5, 7-7, 7-9. Simply circle the attributes applying to you and count the number of circles in each Table. The Table with the most circles is probably your *current* main *dosha*. The Table with the next highest number of circles is your current secondary *dosha*. While this is not necessarily accurate, it will give you an idea of what your *doshas* are now.

Notes

Chapter 8:

The Theory of Relativity: Chinese Medicine

Relativity theory has thus shown that all measurements involving space and time lose their absolute significance and has forced us to abandon the classical concepts of an absolute space and an absolute time.

—Fritjof Capra, physicist[1]

Chinese Medicine is about 4,000 years old. There are many similarities between Chinese Medicine and Ayurveda that leads one to believe Chinese Medicine is derived from Ayurveda. Chinese Medicine does not precisely equate with Ayurvedic terminology, but the foundation of The Five Phases and profound understanding of physics and poetry of Nature is the same.

Chinese Medicine has gone through many changes over the centuries, but it is ancient Classical Chinese Medicine that has been the most valuable to herbal medicine. Herein as we discuss Chinese Medicine, we will be referring to Classical Chinese Medicine unless noted.

The term Traditional Chinese Medicine or TCM came into use when Western medicine began to influence Classical Chinese Medicine after the revolution in 1949. The tendency of TCM trained practitioners is to try to be more "scientific" thereby shifting them to treat more symptomatically. This westernization is essentially what also happened to Western herbal medicine.

There are three fundamental concepts to Chinese Medicine we will discuss that are based on The Five Phases—Yin, Yang, and Qi.

Notes

Yin and Yang and the Theory of Relativity

It is a world of greys, of nuances, of qualifiers, of 'it depends'.
—MATT RIDLEY[2]

The Theory of Yin and Yang, or the dynamic relativity of Nature, is fundamental to Chinese Medicine. All aspects of herbal medicine, diagnosis and treatment, can be summarized and understood in terms of Yin and Yang.

> *The notion of dynamic balance is essential to the way in which the unity of opposites is experienced . . . It is never a static identity, but always a dynamic interplay between two extremes.*
> —FRITJOF CAPRA, PHYSICIST[3]

Yin and Yang can be described in terms of a reference point, where an observer is located, and the perspective from that point, which will be different from another observer's perspective from another reference point. Another way of saying it is that there is no absolute correct interpretation of anything because it depends on your point of view. Everything is relative and depends on your perception.

The concept of Yin and Yang has been restated in Albert Einstein's Special Theory of Relativity. Published in the year 1905, it says that one person's interval of space is not the same as another person's; and time runs at different rates for different observers traveling at different speeds.[4] That is, from where you stand an incident would look different than from where I stand. It took 4,000 years to rediscover Yin and Yang and to restate it in terms of modern physics.

But let's discuss Yin and Yang in a way we can experience it. Yin and Yang are complimentary opposite stages of a process but are always relative to each other and never absolute. For example, night (Yin-time) and day (Yang-time) are always changing. Morning is Yin compared to high noon which is Yang. Evening is Yang compared to the darkest of night. Evening is also Yin compared to daytime. Daytime has the potential to change into the night. Each contains the potential to become its complimentary opposite and transform into each other.

As daytime progresses the Yang of the day is "consumed" or taken over by the Yin of the night and vice versa.

Yin—The Structure

Yin
Moisture of sustenance
Hidden in the shadows
Chill and measured.
Moisture essence
Deep and still
Anchor of life.
—J. SHAMOSH

Notes

Using the foundation of The Five Phases, Yin is comprised of the Phases of Water and Earth. Therefore, Yin has all the properties and effects of these two Phases. (See Chapter 5.)

Yin is the condensed potential energy that we know as matter or substance. It is the static principle relative to Yang.

Table–8-1

THE PHASES & QUALITIES OF YIN

WATER	EARTH
Wet	Heavy
Cold	Dense
Heavy	Solid
Slow	Cold
Dull	Static
Fluid	Nutritious

Yang—The Dynamic Principle

Yang
Rousing the inert
With the vigor of verve
And the sparkle of being
Delighting in the dance
Always seeking the moist
To tame its blaze
And manifest its expression.
—J. Shamosh

Using the foundation of The Five Phases, Yang has all the properties and effects of the Fire Phase. (See Chapter 5.)

Yang as the transforming principle encompasses, but is not limited to, all thermochemical and thermodynamic reactions. It is the compliment of the relatively static and moist Yin.

Table–8-2

THE PHASES & QUALITIES OF YANG

FIRE
Hot
Fluid
Sharp
Light
Clear
Drying
Spreading

Qi—The Transforming Principle

In the discussion of Yin and Yang, only three of The Five Phases were mentioned. To account for the Phases that Yin and Yang do not contain, we have the force known as Qi having the qualities and effects of the Phases of Space and Air. However, Qi seems to also include the concept, from Quantum Theory, of fields and their wave-particles, force and potential energy.

The concept of Qi is as fundamental to Chinese Medicine as Yin and Yang. Qi is the transformational forces, flow, and movement of Nature that allows for the transformation, inter-relationship and interdependence of Yin and Yang.

Since everything began as amorphous energy (or a field of potential), Qi is as subtle and rarefied as the Space and Air Phases and potentially as material as the Earth Phase. In other words when condensed, Qi is physical, and when rarefied, Qi is energy.

In terms of modern physics Qi is the "cosmic dance of energy." Capra states:

> *The particle interactions give rise to the stable structures which build up the material world, which again do not remain static, but oscillate in rhythmic movements. The whole universe is thus engaged in endless motion and activity; in a continual cosmic dance of energy.*[5]

Table–8-3

THE PHASES & EFFECTS OF QI

SPACE	AIR
Rarefied	Movement
Cold	Cold
Movement	Dry
Light	Rough
Clear	Light
Subtle	Clear
Expansive	Subtle

Notes

Notes

Functions of Qi in the Body

Since Qi is as important as Yin and Yang, we will discuss briefly the different qualities of Qi as it relates to the body.

There are many kinds of Qi in the body. Qi can also be deficient or excess. Each organ-system has its own Qi and is relative to, and interdependent on, every other organ-system. For further information see *The Foundations of Chinese Medicine* by Giovanni Maciocia.

The following are the qualities of Qi:

- Transforming, as in metabolic processes of the body.
- Transporting, as in moving food, fluids, and other substances in and out and throughout the body.
- Holding, as in holding fluids and blood in their proper and appropriate places in the body.
- Raising, as in keeping the organs and structures of the body in their proper places.
- Protecting, as in the immune system.
- Warming, as in bodily warmth.

Table–8-4

FUNCTIONS OF QI

Transforming	Metabolic processes
Transporting	Moves food, fluids, substances
Holding	Hold fluids, Blood in pathways
Raising	Holds organs and structures
Protecting	Immune system
Warming	Bodily warmth

The Theory of Yin and Yang

. . . both observer and observed are merging and interpenetrating aspects of one whole reality, which is indivisible and unanalyzable.

—David Bohm, physicist[6]

The most profound description of our world Chinese Medicine has given us is the Theory of Yin and Yang. The Theory of Yin and Yang is based on the duality of experience—hot and cold, up and down, in and out, and so on—and everything is inter-related and interdependent. In modern physics, we can also add particle and wave theory and how they appear to shift back and forth depending on the observer. Everything has both Yin and Yang but in differing proportions. The proportions can also change depending on the situation—relativity and context.

For example, morning-Yang becomes afternoon-Yin. Morning always develops into afternoon. And so, within the Yang-morning, there is always the Yin potential of afternoon waiting for the right conditions to develop. Notice how morning does *not* cause afternoon. There is no cause and effect. The right conditions must develop for afternoon to take place.

The above also illustrates the concept of how everything is relative or interdependent. Afternoon can be either Yin or Yang depending on whether you compare it to morning or night. That is, the degree of Yin or Yang can only be determined relative to something else. Alone it cannot be determined how much Yin or Yang a thing, a substance or person possesses. A thing alone has no value or meaning—no duality for comparison. As physicist David Bohm says, "Opposites are abstract concepts belonging to the realm of thought, and as such they are relative."[7]

Notes

Figure-2

YIN-YANG SYMBOL

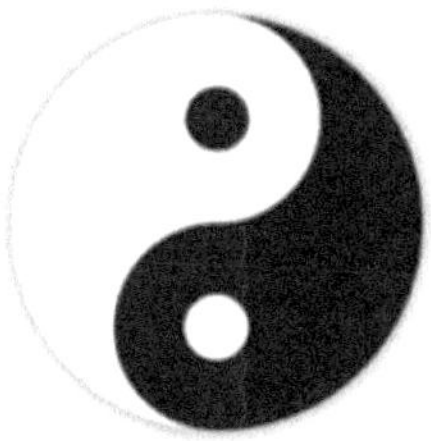

The dots represent the potential of the complimentary opposite quality to manifest in relation to the circumstances. The flowing shape of the Yin and Yang illustrate the ability for one to flow into and become the other also depending on the conditions of relativity.

* * *

The concept behind the Theory of Yin and Yang is also poetically experiential. The best way to understand how Yin and Yang function, their relativity and interdependence, is by using a candle and flame as an example.

The wax making up the candle is the Yin aspect. The candlewax is inert and provides no function unless it is consumed. Once lit with fire or Yang, the candle becomes functional and provides light.

If the flame and the wax of the candle are balanced, we will have enough light for as long as the wax lasts. But, if the wick burns too fast, it quickly consumes the wax and the candle and the light is no more. If the flame is too small, the candle does not provide enough light. Neither extreme is beneficial.

The physical part of our bodies, including our structure—bones, hormones, fluids, enzymes—is the Yin aspect composed of the Phases of Water and Earth. The complement of Yang is that which provides us with thermochemical reactions for metabolism and heat. What animates us, makes us shine, is the Qi aspect made up of the Phases of Space and Air providing for movement and vitality. Our physical bodies would be inert (of no value) without the Yang and the Yang could not be present without the Yin (context) or Qi to keep it dynamically alive.

As with the candle, if we over-stimulate the Yang (flame) it will burn us out too quickly (consume Yin) and we die; but if we do not have enough Yang, we do not have enough energy/Qi to enjoy life. Achieving and maintaining the balance of Yin and Yang is the goal in Chinese Medicine.

Notes

Table–8-5

THE QUALITIES & RELATIVITY OF YIN & YANG

YIN	YANG
Inward	Outward
Downward	Upward
North	South
Dark	Light
Cold	Hot
Heavy	Light
Soft	Hard
Slow	Fast
Peaceful	Restless
Inactive	Active
Wet	Dry
Matter	Energy
Interior	Exterior
Receptive	Aggressive
Feminine	Masculine
Depressed	Excited
Introspective	Extrovert
Particle—Physics	Wave—Physics

Chinese Medicine and Herbal Medicine

The outstanding contribution of Chinese Medicine is its refinement of herbal medicine to the level of high art. The ancient herbal formulations of Chinese Medicine are elegantly, expertly, and logically derived. Many are hundreds to thousands of years old and are extremely effective when applied correctly.

The documentation of the herbs is detailed and precise so the Chinese Medicine herbal practitioner knows what each herb can and will do for a condition and bodily constitution.

However, the descriptions of the effects of Chinese Medicine herbs are in the language of Eastern medicine so foreign to Western minds. One goal of this book is to provide a common language for the Western mind to understand the value and efficacy of Chinese Medicine and Ayurveda by providing Western terminology for the concepts in Eastern medicine.

Yin and Western Society

In Western culture, medical system, institutions, and society, the Yang aspects take precedence and is what is considered and valued. Refer to TABLE 8-5—The Qualities and Relativity of Yin and Yang—and erase all the qualities of Yin; what remains are the qualities of Yang. The rest of your world and experience is missing. You would indeed burn yourself out quickly if there were no rest to balance the activity, no cold to moderate the heat, and so on.

For example, Western trained doctors read numbers on medical tests (Yang information) and compare it to a larger average, but they are not trained to put the information into the context of the individual person whose average may differ from the larger average.

Western society has in fact created an entire race of entities based on the Yang aspect; they are called corporations.

Notes

TABLE–8-6

THE WESTERN PARADIGM

YANG
Outward
Upward
South
Light
Hot
Light
Hard
Fast
Restless
Active
Dry
Energy
Exterior
Aggressive
Male
Excited
Extrovert

Notes

The Balance of Yin and Yang

Another concept unfamiliar to the Western fragmented paradigm is the balance between Yin and Yang and how they support each other. For example, if a person is exhausted, Western medicine usually assumes it is adrenal or thyroid insufficiency and, in some cases, that would be true. However, knowing the erratic and hyperactive lifestyle of Western society, in many cases it is not true. The practitioner of Chinese Medicine looks at the relative balance of Yin and Yang and finds the Yang is sufficient, but the Yin is low and is not *supporting* the Yang.

If this is the case, the remedy in Eastern medicine is to provide herbs/foods to nourish the Yin—herbs containing mostly the Phases of Water and Earth. But, in Western medicine the cure is to administer adrenal hormones and/or thyroid hormones having the effect of further increasing the Yang (stimulating the adrenals or thyroid). Western medicine increases the Yang when the Yin should be increased. In other words, Western medicine would turn up the flame on the candle making the candle burn faster as well as brighter. The supposed cure has then become a poison that consumes the substance (Yin) of the body leaving the system open to side-effects or the mysterious "auto-immune" diseases known in Chinese Medicine as Yin deficiency.

All Western derived medicine has the drawback of being one-sided and Yang oriented regardless of its holistic claims. It is not the fault of only Western medicine; it is pervasive in our mechanistic thinking and is what has created our unbalanced Yang society and institutions.

ILLUSTRATING YIN NOT SUPPORTING YANG

Michelle, a woman in her early 30s, came to see me with extreme tiredness, hair dry and falling out more than usual, and her eyesight was sometimes blurry. She had been to a medical doctor who had done some thyroid tests which came back slightly abnormal. The doctor prescribed thyroid medication.

After the intake and taking her tongue and pulse, I determined she had Liver-System Blood deficiency due to poor eating habits and not enough nourishing food. Michelle was concerned about maintaining her thin figure. In this situation her Blood deficiency (lack of Yin) was causing her Yang-Qi (energy) to be deficient. Thyroid medication, a stimulant, causes one to burn more Yin substance in order to provide energy (think of the flame burning the candlewax) despite a deficient system. What Michelle really needed was more nourishing food to produce nourishing Blood to support her system. Because hair is related to sufficient and nourishing Blood, her hair was dry and falling out more. Her eyes were blurry because the Liver-System, requiring sufficient Blood to function properly, also controls the eyesight.

I counseled her on better food choices and regular eating habits and sent her home with a Chinese herbal formula for Blood deficiency. It took awhile for Michelle to change her eating habits, but she improved. She also stopped the thyroid medication after talking with a pharmacist.

This is a classic case where Yin (Blood) is not supporting the Yang (energy) but she was given a drug that would make her health worse in the long run.

The Systems of the Body in Chinese Medicine

Notes

> *Systems science shows that living systems cannot be understood by analysis . . . The properties of the parts are not intrinsic properties but can be understood only within the context of the larger whole [and so] systems thinking is contextual thinking.*
>
> —Fritjof Capra, physicist[8]

In the Eastern medicine traditions, the body is viewed as being more than the sum of its parts. The body is regarded as an integrated whole—a system of functional relationships and networks integrating bodily functions and fluids, emotions, mental activities, spiritual inclinations, tissues, sense organs, and environmental influences. Because the body is a network of systems within a larger system, the mechanistic anatomical view of medicine does not work. In Eastern medicine, each organ is a complex system functionally inter-related to the other organ-systems, the vital substances, emotions, tissues, and senses. Only through understanding these relationships can an organ-system be defined.

Organ-Systems East and West

The concept of organ-systems in Eastern medicine is a complex network of interrelationships that form a pattern of life. For example, in Western medicine a lung is viewed as a separate part that can be replaced if it is not working properly, like a machine part.

In Eastern medicine, the organ-systems are viewed as a network of functions, interdependent and interrelated with each other. That is, the Lung-System is understood only by its relationships to the other organ-systems and body-context. It is never viewed separate from body, mind, and spirit—the pattern of life. For example, the Lung-System is never discussed by itself. Instead, it is discussed according to its relationships to the other organ-systems, Essential Substances (Blood, Fluids), mind, emotions, and spirit. In turn, these can affect the functions of the Lung-System.

It can take years for the linear and mechanistic mind to become fluent with systems-thinking evident in the complex network and implications of the functions, interactions, and interdependencies of the organ-systems and their processes forming the pattern of life.

Below are some of the intricate interconnections of the body's systems and substances. While the precise and myriad descriptions of the organ-systems and their relationships are beyond the scope of this book, there are many excellent books that can fulfill that requirement. See the bibliography.

Organ-Systems Related to Essential Substances

The organ-systems are interrelated and interdependent on the Essential Substances of Qi, Blood, body Fluids, Essence, and Shen. For example:

Notes

- Heart-System governs the Blood.
- Liver-System stores the Blood.
- Lung-System governs Qi and influences body Fluids.
- Metabolic-System (known as the Spleen in Chinese Medicine) governs Food-Qi, holds Blood in the blood vessels and influences body Fluids.
- Kidney-System stores the Essence and influences body Fluids.

The deficiency or excess of the Essential Substances in turn affect the organ-systems.

Essence

Essence is the basis of our constitutional strength of which there are two sources.

- Innate Essence (Pre-Heaven Essence in Chinese Medicine), genetically derived from our parents, determines each person's unique constitution, physiological strength and vitality.
- Daily Essence (Post-Heaven Essence in Chinese Medicine) is extracted by the Lung-System from the air we breathe and by the Metabolic-System from the foods we eat and the fluids we drink. Therefore, quality food, drink, and air are of vital importance to our health.

The combination of the two Essences, that are "located" in the Kidney-System, determines growth, reproduction, development, sexual maturation, conception, pregnancy, menopause, and ageing. If Essence is consumed by poor lifestyle choices it can be replaced but only with a great deal of effort.

Innate Essence + Daily Essence = Kidney Essence

Blood

Blood is derived from several combined sources. The energy we extract from our food and drink (Food-Qi) produced by the Metabolic-System is combined with the energy from the air we breathe (Air-Qi) and then also combined with the Qi of the Heart-System (Heart-Qi) and then transformed into Blood.

Blood nourishes with both nutrients and Qi, moistens the tissues of the body, is the foundation for Shen (Mind-Heart-Spirit, discussed later), and is closely interrelated to Essence and Fluids (discussed later).

Food-Qi + Air-Qi + Heart-Qi = Blood

Fluids

The body Fluids originate from our food and drink (Food-Qi) and then transformed by intricate purification processes by the Metabolic-System.

Notes

The Essential Fluids are closely interrelated to Blood, Qi and Essence. Essential Fluids moisten the joints, membranes, skin, muscles, and other tissues and structures of the body.

Food-Qi + Metabolic-System = Essential Fluids

Shen (Heart-Mind)

Shen is the combination of the mind, emotions (Heart and Liver-Systems), and the spirit (that "resides" in the Heart-System). Shen is the complicated emotional response-pattern of a person's personality. Shen, the Heart-Mind, is the mental-emotional aspect of the peptide communication network of the body affecting the response-pattern the body will then manifest.

Shen influences all the manifestations of the functions of our bodies but mainly determines our perception, memory, sleep, feelings, and the senses.

Mind + Emotions + Spirit (Heart-Mind) = Shen

Organ-Systems Related to Tissues

There is a functional relationship between the tissues of the body and each organ-system. Observing the corresponding tissue will help to determine the state of health of the organ-system. For example, the complexion will tell us the state of the Heart-System. The degree of flexibility of the sinews and condition of the nails gives us insight to the Liver-System. The condition of the skin and body hair gives information about the Lung-System. The muscles and lips inform us about the Metabolic-System. The bones and head hair tell us about the Kidney-System.

TABLE–8-7

ORGAN-SYSTEMS & TISSUES

ORGAN-SYSTEM	TISSUE
Heart	Complexion color
Liver	Sinews, nails
Lung	Skin, body hair
Metabolic	Muscles, lip color
Kidney	Bones, head hair

Organ-Systems Related to Sense Organs

There is a functional relationship between each organ-system and each of the sense organs. The health and acuity of a sense organ relies on the adequate nourishment of its corresponding organ-system. For example, the Heart-System controls the tongue and taste; the

Notes

Liver-System controls the eyes and sight; the Lung-System controls the nose and smell; the Metabolic-System controls the mouth and taste; the Kidney-System controls the ears and hearing.

Table–8-8

ORGAN-SYSTEMS & SENSE ORGANS

ORGAN-SYSTEM	SENSE ORGAN
Heart	Tongue, taste
Liver	Eyes, sight
Lung	Nose, smell
Metabolic	Mouth, taste
Kidney	Ears, hearing

Organ-Systems Related to Emotions

In Eastern medicine, the emotions determine the responses of the organ-systems. Therefore, the state of an organ-system will affect the emotions and vice versa. For example, the Heart-System relates to joy or sadness, the Liver-System relates to anger; the Lung-System relates to grief and worry; the Metabolic-System relates to thinking; the Kidney-System relates to fear. When an emotion is excessive, repressed, or prolonged it will create an imbalance in the corresponding organ-system. Therefore, treating the organ-system can influence the emotions and help restore balance.

The idea that only the mind can affect the body is a one-sided view because the body can also affect the mind as seen in Eastern medicines. Eugene Wigner (1902-1995), a Nobel Prize winning physicist stated that "if mind could not affect the physical world but was only affected by it, this would be the only known example in modern physics of such a one-way interaction. For in modern physics one-way interactions are not known to occur."[9]

Table–8-9

ORGAN-SYSTEMS & EMOTIONS

ORGAN-SYSTEM	EMOTION
Heart	Joy, sadness
Liver	Anger
Lung	Grief, worry
Metabolic	Thinking
Kidney	Fear

Organ-Systems Related to the Environment

Notes

The organ-systems are influenced by the environment, climate, and weather since we are made of the same substances. Excessive or prolonged exposure to extremes of these can adversely affect the organ-systems. For example, heat will influence the Heart-System; wind will influence the Liver-System; dryness will influence the Lung-System; dampness will influence the Metabolic-System; cold will influence the Kidney-System.

Table–8-10

ORGAN-SYSTEMS & ENVIRONMENT

ORGAN-SYSTEM	ENVIRONMENT
Heart	Heat
Liver	Wind
Lungs	Dryness
Metabolic	Dampness
Kidney	Cold

Table–8-11

ORGAN-SYSTEMS RELATIONSHIPS

ORGAN-SYSTEM	TISSUE	SENSE ORGAN	EMOTION	ENVIRONMENT
Heart	Complexion color	Tongue, taste	Joy, sadness	Heat
Liver	Sinews, nails	Eyes, sight	Anger	Wind
Lung	Skin, body hair	Nose, smell	Grief, worry	Dryness
Metabolic	Muscles, lip color	Mouth, taste	Thinking	Dampness
Kidney	Bones, head hair	Ears, hearing	Fear	Cold

Part Three:

Fusion Systems of Herbal Medicine

Notes

Chapter 9:

Unified Systems of Ayurveda & Chinese Medicine

Disease is seen in a context—a milieu of behavior, diet, sleep and exercise patterns, and various other relationships with the world at large . . . as part of a process of living which can accurately be described as an unbroken whole.

—Larry Dossey, M.D.[1]

Since Classical Chinese Medicine seems to be derived from Ayurveda, there are more similarities between the two than there are differences. Ayurveda emphasizes the appropriate foods and routines of daily life and mental and spiritual health of the individual to maintain the flowing balance in the body. Chinese Medicine is most noted for its precise documentation of herbs and their actions and detailed explanations of the body systems functions and interrelationships. That is not to say that Classical Chinese Medicine believes that daily lifestyle and mental and spiritual aspects are unimportant, but it is emphasized less in most current practices. That is also not to say that Ayurveda does not have a rich history of herbal medicine and documentation.

Ayurveda's Clinical Excellence

The value of understanding and determining the constitution-context of a person in Ayurveda gives the Systems Herbalist unparalleled insight into, not only the person's current physical condition, but mental, emotional, and spiritual tendencies. This insight is most helpful in determining, not only the probable origin of their imbalance and what

Notes

questions to ask the person for detail, but also the herbs that are needed, or avoided, to bring the person back into their unique flowing balance.

By knowing the original-constitution and the unbalanced-state of the person, the Systems Herbalist can counsel and advise the person correctly. The Systems Herbalist will know what to say and how to say it so the person will not respond with disregard or resistance and will be more likely to follow the lifestyle guidelines presented.

For example, Vata-people tend to have erratic lifestyles. They can only manage to change one or two things at a time. Knowing this, the Systems Herbalist can prioritize the needed changes but only ask for one or two changes at a time, such as getting to bed earlier, or eating on a regular schedule. If the Systems Herbalist were to list all the needed changes at once, the Vata-person would be overwhelmed, will fail to improve and may not return.

Pitta-people tend to become resistant when the Systems Herbalist asks for lifestyle changes. Instead, the Systems Herbalist should encourage the Pitta-person's willingness to cooperate by *asking* the Pitta-person if they would be willing to make a change if it would help them feel better. Then the Systems Herbalist needs to explain to the Pitta-person *why* the change is being requested.

Kapha-people tend to inertia and will, therefore, need encouragement to change, but once they start, they are faithful and compliant people. Lack of adequate exercise, improper diet, and poor digestion is usually the Kapha-person's underlying problem. The Systems Herbalist should find out what the Kapha-person likes to do that involves movement and give them concrete ideas on how to eat better for their constitution and condition.

Ayurveda and Pulse Diagnosis

The detail available in Ayurvedic pulse diagnosis is beyond compare and very accurate once mastered. The pulse is felt at seven levels on the radial artery of both wrists, under six fingertips, and three to five points on each fingertip. Upon reading the Ayurvedic pulse of a person, the Systems Herbalist can determine what *dosha*s are predominant and out of balance and in which organ-systems and/or tissues. As such, the Systems Herbalist will know whether to treat for the pathogenic (capable of producing disease) factors of wind, cold, damp, dry, or heat and combinations thereof. In addition, the Ayurvedic pulse tells the Systems Herbalist in what tissues (plasma, blood, muscle, fat, bone, nerve, and reproductive) the problem is occurring. This information can be accessed in the Chinese Medicine pulse but with more subjectivity and therefore less accuracy.

Notes

Chinese Medicine's Clinical Excellence

Chinese Medicine gives the Systems Herbalist another method to confirm a diagnosis similar to having a second opinion.

Once the diagnosis is confirmed in Chinese Medicine terms (See Chapter 12), the person is advised how they can participate in their healing by adjusting their lifestyle. Then the Systems Herbalist decides on an herbal treatment until the person is to be seen again. The next time the person is seen s/he may present differently, and the herbal treatment may need to be changed. Since the body is a flowing system, the Systems Herbalist should assume the person may present differently each time they are seen.

Chinese herbal medicine is a high art that has been passed down to us over thousands of years. Used properly, Chinese herbal medicine is amazingly precise, effective, and fast acting. In fact, people can feel changes within a few minutes of taking liquid herbal formulas.

The key is to be able to either find the correct herbal formula or to compose your own (See Chapter 12). Since there are thousands of ancient formulations available in books, most often the Systems Herbalist can find or modify a formula to suit the need. Many years of learning the formulas and herbs, along with great skill, are needed to prescribe the correct formula. Apprenticing with someone who has at least ten years of experience is recommended.

Chinese Medicine Pulse Diagnosis

Chinese Medicine pulse diagnosis is essential to learn as it is in Ayurveda otherwise the Systems Herbalist relies on the Western diagnosis or symptoms for treatment. The Western diagnosis tells us about the disease but nothing about the person who has the disease or condition. Treating the disease is treating symptoms, as opposed to treating the person's response-pattern, and is to be strictly avoided.

Chinese Medicine pulse diagnosis can be very accurate. It is felt at 3 to 4 levels on the radial artery of both wrists, under six fingertips and relies on the subjective interpretation of the 28 different qualities that the pulse can exhibit at each level. It takes many years to master the Chinese Medicine pulse as it does the Ayurvedic pulse.

Tongue Diagnosis

Tongue diagnosis is used in both Ayurveda and Chinese Medicine. Tongue diagnosis is an accurate and helpful tool but generally does not give enough detailed information about deeper conditions. It is helpful to assess the tongue first as it will give information that can help the Systems Herbalist look in certain areas of the pulse to see where an imbalance may lie.

Notes

FIGURE–3

TONGUE DIAGNOSIS CHART

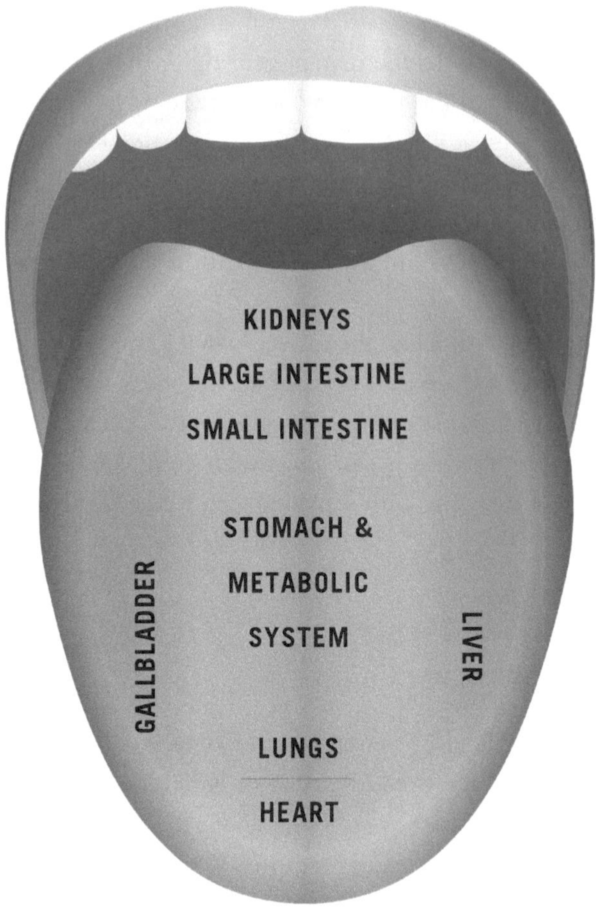

Ayurvedic and Chinese Medicine Terminology

Using deductive reasoning, we will discuss specifically how the terminology of Ayurveda and Chinese Medicine integrate and how they can be used together to achieve a better understanding of each person and their disorder.

The Five Phases are essential to understanding how Ayurveda and Chinese Medicine correlate since this is the foundation of both remarkable and effective forms of medicine.

In the following, we will discuss the doshas of Ayurveda and correlate them with Chinese Medicine terminology.

Vata & Chinese Medicine

Notes

The Phases of Space and Air in Ayurveda compose the Vata principle. In Chinese Medicine, these Phases are associated with the concept of Qi, except Qi often includes the quality of Heat, which is unlike Vata, who tends to be cold. Therefore, using the term deficient from Chinese Medicine with a tendency to coldness (as in deficient Qi), coincides with the rarefied nature of Vata due to Space and Air Phases, which are also cold.

Deficient = Rarefied/Cold (Space & Air)

The additional quality of cold is necessary to account for the reduced heat in the Vata system due to the Space and Air Phases.

Adding the term Yin, we have the Chinese Medicine term deficient-Yin that refers to the lack of Essential Fluids or dryness that correlates with the dry quality of Vata.

Deficient Yin = Dry

Therefore,

Vata = Deficient Yin-Cold
or
Rarefied, Dry, Cold

Pitta & Chinese Medicine

The next Phases are Fire and Water. In Ayurveda, these Phases together are Pitta. In Chinese Medicine, these same Phases would be Yang. These two terms are easily reconciled as they are near equivalents in describing the heat and transforming aspects of both Pitta and Yang. The Water Phase in Yang is assumed as some water is required to moderate the heat or all substance would be transformed into energy.

Pitta = Yang
or
Heat

Kapha & Chinese Medicine

The next Phases are Water and Earth. In Ayurveda, these Phases are Kapha. In Chinese Medicine, the Water and Earth Phases would be Yang deficiency or lack of sufficient heat and the quality of cold.

Yang Deficiency = Cold

Notes

However, it is not quite equivalent as Kapha is also wet. Yang deficient describes the coldness of Kapha. The addition of the term wet accounts for the Water Phase or damp and heavy qualities of Kapha.

Kapha = Yang Deficient-Wet
or
Cold, Wet, Heavy

Vata = Deficient Yin-Cold

Pitta = Yang

Kapha = Yang Deficient-Wet

Table–9-1

AYURVEDA & CHINESE MEDICINE UNIFIED

PHASES	AYURVEDA	CHINESE MEDICINE	QUALITIES
Space & Air	Vata	Deficient Yin-Cold	Rarefied, Dry, Cold
Fire & Water	Pitta	Yang	Heat
Water & Earth	Kapha	Yang deficient-Wet	Cold, Wet, Heavy

Table–9-2

EQUATING AYURVEDA & CHINESE MEDICINE TERMINOLOGY

AYURVEDA	CHINESE MEDICINE
Vata (constitution)	Deficient-Yin-Cold
Pitta (constitution)	Yang
Kapha (constitution)	Yang-Deficient-Wet
Vata	Qi
Vata Pushing Pitta	Yin-Deficiency
Agni	Metabolic-System (Spleen)
Ama	Phlegm
Ojas	Essence
Kapha	Fluids
Ahamkara	Shen

Notes

Chapter 10:

Macrocosmic & Microcosmic Climates

The behavior of microscopic components reverberates to the macroscopic level.

—Larry Dossey, M.D.[1]

Climate and weather are something everyone has experienced because we live in the conditions created daily. Therefore, describing bodily conditions in terms of internal weather renders The Five Phases and their attributes understandable in a more experiential way. These different climatic conditions capable of invading the body are called pathogenic (capable of producing disease) factors in Eastern medicine.

Weather—External and Internal

One can easily feel the effects of the weather changing from hot to cool, cold to warm, windy to calm, calm to stormy, dry to rainy etc. The results of climate and weather changes in the external environment or macrocosm, have the same effect in the internal microcosm of the body. This creates internal conditions for which we have terms not usually associated with weather or climate changes. For example, an internal condition of too much mucus would be described as damp and wet weather internally.

The environment is essential to consider when administering herbs/foods because the environment also exhibits the attributes of The Five Phases affecting our bodies. For example, the environment in the southwest (USA) is hot and dry with the predominant Phases of Air and Fire. In this climate, the herbal practitioner would be careful to not additionally dry and warm Vata-Pitta constitution persons because the environment is already drying

Notes

and warming. Likewise, when administering herbs/foods to Kapha constitution in a cool and damp climate, such as the northwest (USA), caution is needed to avoid making them more cold and wet internally. The concept of the larger macrocosm affecting our internal microcosm is illustrated in TABLE-10-1 AND 10-2.

Of course, in any of these climates you can have daily weather changes. For example, when it rains in the Southwest, the normal dry and warm conditions can turn to wet and cold temporarily.

Seasons and Internal Microcosm

There are also different seasons influencing our internal microcosm. Spring and fall are times of change from either winter to summer or summer to winter. Because of the changing environment, these seasons are often windy exhibiting the Phases of Space and Air.

The Vata constitution can have more problems in the spring and fall due to their predominant Air Phase and subsequent sensitivity to weather changes. Some of the changes that can affect Vata constitution during this season are dryness, coldness, constipation, variable digestion and appetite, tiredness, insomnia, abdominal distention, stiffness, tremors, and twitches. (See Chapter 7.)

Summer would adversely affect Pitta constitution due to the predominant Fire Phase of the season. Pitta constitution may exhibit skin inflammations, rashes, loose stools, excessive hunger and thirst, burning sensations, sleeplessness, feverishness, and excessive perspiration. (See Chapter 7.)

Fall is also a time of change affecting Vata constitution. However, Pitta constitution may also be affected from the accumulation of heat during the summer.

Winter can adversely affect Kapha constitution due to cold and often wet conditions from the Water Phase. If Kapha constitution is out of balance, there could be a loss of strength and stamina, flaccidity, susceptibility to colds, mucus and/or phlegm congestion and accumulation, obesity, excessive sleeping, dullness, coldness, water retention, inertia, high blood sugar, and respiratory problems. (See Chapter 7.)

Table–10-1

CLIMATE: MICROCOSM/MACROCOSM

** Conditions are potential pathogenic factors*

PHASES	AYURVEDA	CHINESE MEDICINE	CONDITIONS	CLIMATE	SEASON
Space & Air	Vata	Deficient Yin-Cold	Rarefied	Alaska	Spring
Fire & Water	Pitta	Yang	Hot, Damp	Southeast, USA	Summer
Water & Earth	Kapha	Yang-Deficient-Wet	Cold, Damp, Heavy	Northwest, USA	Winter
Air & Fire	Vata-Pitta	Yin-Deficiency-Fire	Dry, Hot	Southwest, USA	Summer

Notes

Chapter 11:

Person-Condition Relativity

All the systems concepts discussed so far can be seen as different aspects of one great strand as systemic thinking, which we may call contextual thinking.

—Fritjof Capra, physicist[1]

To arrive at a correct diagnosis, the herbal practitioner must be able to identify the current condition of the person-context relative to the disorder *within* the person, also known as the root-cause. The Eight Principles help to qualify the information in relation to person-context, where the disharmony is located, as well as determining the disorder. This information helps to identify and address a condition *before* it becomes a disease pattern.

The Eight Principles of Herbal Medicine

The Eight Principles come to us from Chinese Medicine and are the dualities of Yin and Yang, Excess and Deficiency, Hot and Cold, Interior and Exterior. The Eight Principles is the process of classifying the person-context and the disorder.

Each category is relative. In other words, it is not wholly Yin or Yang, Excess or Deficient but interrelated and can include both at times. For example, one may have an excess condition in one area and a deficient condition in another area. In addition, not all categories of the Eight Principles will fit every situation. For example, not all disharmonies involve hot or cold conditions.

Notes

ILLUSTRATING DEFICIENT AND EXCESS

If the Kidney Yang is deficient, there is often coldness of the lower extremities because the Kidney-System, besides being cold, cannot hold the heat in the lower body. Therefore, the upper body may be relatively more hot. This can be compared to a fireplace and chimney where the damper is wide open allowing all the heat to escape upwards leaving the room cold. In this scenario we would give an herbal formula that would "anchor the Yang" effectively closing the damper so the heat does not escape upwards and perhaps also use herbs to extinguish the upward draft of wind.

Exterior and Interior

Exterior and interior refer to the location of the disharmony. We want to know where in the body the condition lies because the subsequent treatment will be different; that is, the relationship of the disorder in the person can differ according to the location of the disorder.

Exterior

Exterior refers to the Lung-System, skin and muscles, and the areas between the skin and muscles. It is associated with the first level of the immune system and is the first area attacked by an airborne pathogen and other environmental factors such as Wind. (The Lung-System is always in contact with the exterior environment.)

The symptoms of an Exterior condition are acute onset, such as a cold/flu. This condition will be further differentiated according to Hot or Cold and Excess or Deficient to determine the treatment strategy.

Depending on the hot or cold exterior condition, Herbs That Release the Surface would be used to help move the pathogenic factor out of the body; like opening windows in a house to air it out.

Interior

Interior refers to the inside of the body and the organ-systems, Qi, Blood-System, or Fluids. Even though an external condition, such as a cold or flu, begins in the exterior, once it penetrates to the interior, it is considered an interior condition and would be treated differently than if it were in the exterior level.

An interior condition can cause harm to the interior systems and develop into a disease-pattern if not treated properly. For example, heat and wind in the Blood-System can cause itchy and red skin disorders; heat damaging the Fluids can cause Yin-deficiency and develop into an auto-immune disorder. The herbs used would vary greatly depending on the condition and the person.

Notes

Hot and Cold

The duality of hot and cold refers to the degree of heat (or lack of heat) that is present in a person compared to the relative hot or cold of the condition. The presence of heat or cold would be further qualified by Excess or Deficiency.

For example, excess heat can be due to a fever or inflammation or simply an overheated condition. Or, one may have a deficiency of heat, such as shivering, or excess cold with extreme symptoms of coldness in the body, such as persistent chills or hypothermia.

There can also be combined Hot and Cold, such as Heat in the upper body and Cold in the lower body or Cold in the Exterior and Heat in the Interior.

Hot

Heat in the system can be either Excess or Deficient.

Excess-heat can be External or Internal. Internal Excess-heat presents with symptoms such as sensations of heat or burning, thirst, restlessness, red colorations such as red face or rash, among other indications.

Deficient-heat usually refers to deficiency of Yin usually in one or more organs-systems. Generally, the symptoms are feelings of heat late in the day and at night (Yin time of day), dry throat at night, scanty and/or dark yellow urine, among other symptoms. This will be discussed further under Yin.

Cold

Cold in the body can be either Excess or Deficient.

Excess-cold presents with feelings of cold or aversion to cold, little or no thirst, pale coloration, abundant and colorless urine, among other symptoms.

Deficient-cold is due to the deficiency of Yang or not enough heat. The symptoms are feeling cold and aversion to cold, dull and pale complexion, poor digestion, loose stools, tiredness, weakness, among other symptoms.

Excess and Deficiency

The determination of Excess and Deficiency in diagnosis involves evaluating the person's constitutional strength relative to the presence or lack of a pathogenic factor—Wind, Cold, Heat Dampness, or Dryness—and the strength of the pathogenic factor itself.

Excess

An Excess condition is determined by the presence of a pathogenic factor where the body's strength or Qi is strong enough to be able to fight off the pathogenic factor.

Excess conditions usually come on quickly and present with irritability, restlessness, pain aggravated by pressure, heavy breathing, among other symptoms.

Notes

Deficiency

A Deficiency condition is where the body's Qi is not strong and there is no pathogenic factor present. There can be deficiency of Qi, Blood, Yin or Yang.

Deficiency conditions usually present with tiredness, and weakness and more depending on the organ-system or Essential Substance being affected.

Excess with Deficiency

This is a combination pattern where the body's Qi is too deficient to respond sufficiently or effectively to the stronger, excess pathogenic factor that is present.

Yin and Yang

The duality of Yin and Yang was discussed in detail in Chapter 8 on Chinese Medicine. In this context, The Eight Principles use the concept of relativity or proportion of the other six Principles when referring to Yin and Yang. The other situations where the Principle of Yin and Yang are used are in cases of the Deficiency of Yin, discussed below, or the extreme of deficiency called collapse of Yin or Yang, but these will not be discussed here.

Yin-Deficiency

An important concept in Chinese Medicine is Yin-deficiency. Yin-deficiency refers to the lack of Yin or Essential Fluids in the body presenting with symptoms, such as dryness in the joints or insufficient hormones. When there is insufficient moisture in the body to moderate the heat or Yang, the body feels too hot and has the potential to consume itself or burn itself out. It is as if the flame of the candle is too big and is consuming the wax too fast eventually extinguishing the candle.

The condition of Yin-Deficiency can be confusing to Westerners because it *appears* there is excess heat or inflammation in the body. Though the outward symptoms seem the same, there is a significant difference between Yin-deficiency and excess heat. With the condition of excess heat, the body truly contains too much heat. With the condition of Yin-deficiency, the essential bodily Fluids are low resulting in the relative appearance of too much heat. Incorrect treatment will make the person worse.

Comparing Yin-deficiency to a car engine: the car may be running hot because there is not enough coolant in the system as opposed to the car running hot from overwork. If you treated your coolant-deficient car by giving it more gasoline, the problem of overheating would continue. Eventually the chronic condition of lack of coolant would cause the engine to get so hot it would seize up and no longer function.

In Western medicine, the coolant-deficient car may present in a person with the appearance of adrenal deficiency because there may be sluggishness or tiredness due to the system being out of balance—insufficient Yin to support the Yang. Indeed, there is a deficiency but not of the Yang (heat) systems. What is needed is more coolant in terms of Yin Fluids but what is often administered is more gasoline to keep the engine running. In other words, the person is given more stimulant in the form of adrenal or thyroid

Notes

hormones serving to advance the condition more quickly. Eventually the system burns itself out.

Yin-deficiency is the source of many auto-immune diseases becoming rampant in our overly Yang and imbalanced society. Auto-immune disorders are considered incurable because of the inability of Western medicine to recognize, and therefore treat, the concept of Yin in its deficiency state. Auto-immune diseases are correctly described as the body consuming itself (the large flame consuming the wax too fast) but the cause and correct treatment is not known to Western medicine because it is unaware of the concepts of Yin and Yin-deficiency.

Figure–4

EXCESS & DEFICIENT YIN & YANG

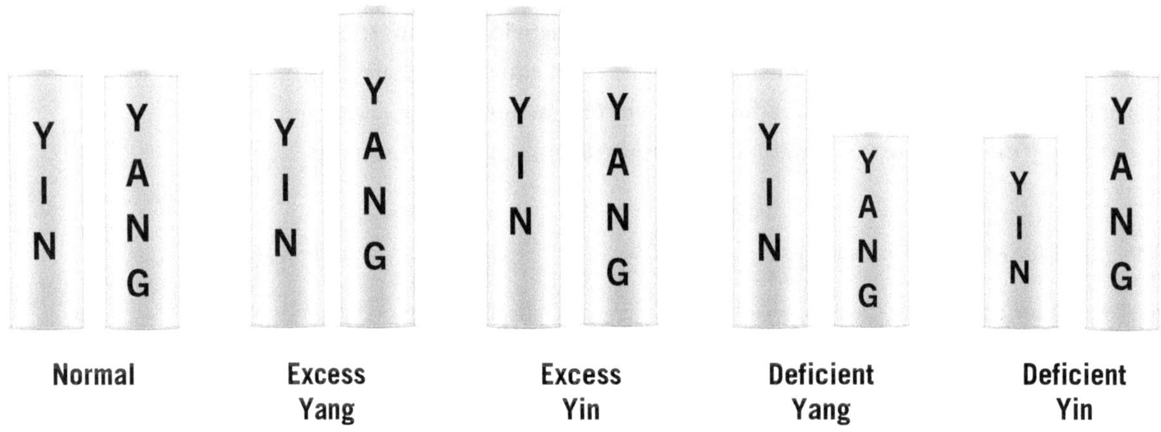

Excess Yang and Deficient Yin both will feel hot but for different reasons. Excess Yang has too much Yang compared to normal Yin. Deficient Yin has too little Yin compared to a normal Yang. These very different situations present the same but are treated very differently in Eastern medicine. In comparison, Western medicine, unaware of Yin, treats Deficient Yin as if it were Deficient Yang resulting in more heat which in turn further reduces the Yin.

Notes

Chapter 12:

Systems Treatment in Herbal Medicine

It is in becoming whole that we become well.
—J. Shamosh

The aspiring Systems Herbalist should have a comprehensive systems-based foundation to avoid resorting to symptoms. In Eastern medicine, the Systems Herbalist must:

I. First, master **PRINCIPLES BEFORE STRATEGIES** such as The Functional Principles Theory and The Five Phases as discussed in the previous chapters, to avoid resorting to symptoms and diagnosing diseases.

II. Second, master **SYSTEMS-TREATMENT** strategies, which will be discussed in this chapter, and is based on the systems of The Functional Principles and The Five Phases. This can only be learned in a clinical setting.

III. Third, master **HERBAL FORMULA CATEGORIES** discussed in this chapter.

IV. Learn the **SPECIFIC HERBS** that make up the formulas which will be discussed in following chapters.

It is up to the Systems Herbalist to determine the person's unhealthy patterns *before* they manifest as a response-pattern. For example: treat uprising wind-phlegm before it manifests or it can result in a wind-stroke. It is why the ancient Chinese herbal practitioner was only paid when the person was healthy. If the person got sick, it was because the practitioner did not detect an unhealthy pattern developing.

Notes

Label a person's pattern (diagnosis) for that moment only keeping in mind that it can change by the next time you see them. If you have used the correct strategy and herbal formula(s), you should see a different presentation in the next visit. Therefore, never expect the same presentation or the same diagnosis on subsequent visits. Try to change the system-response so that the unhealthy pattern will also change.

The Four Observations

Carefully observing the person is extremely important because it gives the practitioner information on the person-context that has the condition.

1. **Seeing**—notice demeanor, dry or oily hair, nails, skin coloration, energy/qi level, agitation, quietness, etc.
2. **Hearing**—listening to the sound and pitch of the voice, breathing, abdominal sounds, sighing, a cough, or other sounds.
3. **Smelling**—different odors relate to different problems, such as bad breath in stomach problems or strong body odor in Liver-System conditions.
4. **Asking**—questioning to diagnose and confirm a pattern. Find out how and when the problem arose, work and living environment, family issues, sleep, elimination, etc.

Use a Questionnaire

A questionnaire can be used to get a general idea of what the conditions may be, but a questionnaire is *not a substitute* for the above observations. If there is a medical diagnosis, determine the acute pattern[s] that may be present by translating the diagnosis into Eastern medicine. For example: arthritis can be wind-damp; wind-cold, wind-cold-damp, wind-heat, wind-heat-damp, etc.

Sometimes the medical diagnosis is a label that includes many different patterns of the same disease. For example: high blood pressure can have 75 or more different combinations of patterns and diabetes at least 20 different combinations of patterns.

If there is no medical diagnosis, determine what unhealthy patterns may be present. Sometimes the medical treatment is the cause of the condition, in which case, the Systems Herbalist needs to know the actions of the different pharmaceuticals in Eastern medicine terms. This can be determined by knowing the side-effects of the drug.

Tongue Assessment

Tongue assessment is used to determine what generally may be happening in the system. The practitioner should notice the tongue body and coating or lack of coating, thickness, color, and location of the coating; features of the tongue, moisture or lack of moisture, color of the tongue body, movement, or short/long tongue.

Notes

ILLUSTRATING SYSTEMS DIAGNOSIS AND TREATMENT

Shirley worked in a doctor's office for many years when she was referred to me. She came in, sat down and said, "I don't believe in what you do but I have no where else to go." She then told me she has a large and deep abscess on her leg that is not responding to treatment and the doctors want to cut out a large portion of her leg that would leave her permanently lame.

I proceeded to do an intake, and near the end, when I go over foods eaten, I asked her if she drank coffee and how much. Her answer was that she drank 8-10 pots of coffee a day. Thinking she meant 8-10 cups, I asked her again. When she said pots, I repeated the word in disbelief.

Her tongue and pulses indicated damp-heat toxin. I asked her if any of the many doctors she saw ever asked what she put in her mouth. She said no. I then asked her if she would be willing to stop drinking coffee and eliminate acidic foods (Pitta food guidelines. See www.ayurveda.com). She said she would if it meant saving her leg. I gave her a Chinese herbal formula to clear damp-heat toxin and sent her home.

When she returned two weeks later, it was with a big smile on her face. She said the abscess was almost gone. By the way, I never saw the abscess!

The abscess was just the symptom of a problem brought on by improper lifestyle, in this case, poor food choices. Treating the underlying root cause of damp-heat-toxin solved the cause and the system-response, also damp-heat-toxin. Even if the doctors could have eliminated the abscess/symptom, the cause would still be in her system and would have eventually created another condition that would possibly have been worse.

Pulse Assessment

Pulse assessment is used to determine which pathogenic factors are present and how they are affecting the general system, organ-systems, or how the organ-systems are affecting each other. Therefore, determine which relationships within the system are healthy (strengths) or unhealthy relationships (weaknesses). For example: Liver-System invading Metabolic-System pattern or uprising wind-phlegm pattern.

Based on the assessment, determine the treatment strategy according to what needs to be accomplished for the person to improve. For example: if the assessment is Liver-System invading the Metabolic-System then regulating the Liver-System will stop that pattern; or if there is excess wind and phlegm, reducing wind and transforming phlegm will alleviate the pattern. Notice how the diagnosis leads to the correct strategy.

Root and Response-Pattern

In Eastern medicine, the manifestation of the disorder (symptom) is treated only in the context of the person's unique response-pattern along with the *Energetic* nature and location of the

Notes

disorder.[1] "Treatment in Eastern medicine is not disorder-oriented (linear cause and effect), but is strategy or systems-oriented. The treatment strategy in turn is based on the underlying cause [root] of a disease."[2] That is, the treatment strategy is inseparable from the diagnostics.

For example, in the case of an invading flu/cold, we want to know about the environment of the person who has the virus and what that virus is doing to the person's system in order to survive. If it is a virus that likes a cold internal climate (microcosm) to live in, then we would change the internal climate so the virus could no longer survive. In other words, we would warm the internal environment of the person. This would eliminate the virus because it could no longer exist in the warmer climate. This strategy is confirmed by microbiologist Rene Dubois (1901-1982) who stated, "Most microbial diseases are caused by organisms present in the body of a normal individual. They become the cause of disease when a disturbance arises which upsets the equilibrium of the body."[3]

A diagnosed disorder can also be treated in different ways depending on The Functional Principles involved. For example, a digestive disorder involving bloating and gas can be rooted in a deficient (cold) Metabolic-System or rooted in an excess (heat) pattern due to stagnation of energy/qi in the Liver-System adversely affecting the Metabolic-System. These very different roots, of the apparently same response-pattern, would be treated very differently. To treat them the same would cause one person to get better and the other one to get worse.

It takes many years of clinical training and experience to accurately assess the difference between the root and the response-pattern of a disorder as well as to determine which is foremost to be treated.

* * *

ILLUSTRATING SYSTEMS DIAGNOSIS AND TREATMENT

A father and teenage son came to see me. The father was a student at the naturopathic college (Western-based training) where I occasionally lectured. The son, obviously in distress, had a condition where his abdomen was constantly and painfully cramping making him unable to stand up straight. Over the past month the concerned father had brought him to many different doctors, including a gastro-intestinal specialist, a nephrologist and several others who had all done their various tests, with no conclusive results.

I looked at his tongue and took his pulses and determined he had cold-damp in the middle (mid-section of the body which includes the Stomach, Metabolic, and Liver Systems). I gave him ¼ teaspoon of a warming and spasm relieving Ayurvedic powdered formula followed by water. Within a few seconds, he took a deep breath, stood up straight and smiled. The father's eyes became huge with amazement. After a month of taking his son to all kinds of doctors who only read test results, what worked was a small amount of the right herbal formula that fixed the son's mysterious problem.

Notes

Originally, in Chapter 3, it was said that root and response-pattern in Eastern medicine are the same, and they are when viewing the person-context. However, we can break these concepts down for the benefit of treatment strategy as follows:

- The strength of the person's constitution (context) is the root, and the relative strength of the individual principles involved, from The Functional Principles, of the invading pathogen (factors of heat, cold, dry, damp, wind) is the response-pattern.
- The cause of the disorder (invading pathogenic factors of heat, cold, dry, damp, wind) is the root *and* the response-pattern.
- During the ailment, the primary disorder is the root and any secondary complications are response-pattern.
- The location (Organ-System, tissue, or channel) of a disorder, if internal is the root, if external is the response-pattern.
- If a disorder is acute, treat the response-pattern.
- If a disorder is chronic, treat the root.[4]

Simultaneous treatment of root and response-pattern are where:

- The person's constitutional strength needs to be supported at the same time the invading pathogen needs to be eliminated.
- Where there are false symptoms, as in Yin-deficiency, where the false symptom of heat (response-pattern) would be cleared while the Yin (context) would be supported.[5]

Because the diagnosis and herbal treatment strategies are the same in Eastern herbal medicine, listed here are the herbal formulas in categories according to Bensky and Barolet's *Formulas & Strategies.* The purpose here is to translate some Eastern medicine concepts and introduce the categories of herbal formulas in order to familiarize the Western herbalist or medical doctor with the Eastern strategies of treatment that work so well. This is not a comprehensive explanation of the categories. For more detailed information and further study, please refer to Bensky and Barolet's *Chinese Herbal Medicine Formulas & Strategies* in the bibliography.

There are no standard herbal formulas in Western herbal medicine, only categories of herbs, which will be discussed in Chapter 14. However, the following tables correlate the Eastern categories of formulas from *Chinese Herbal Medicine Formulas & Strategies* with the categories of Western herbs as much as possible. There are many overlapping Western categories due to non-differentiation of The Functional Principles of the herbs in Western herbal medicine.

Notes

Table–12-1

CATEGORIES OF FORMULAS: HERBS

Eastern Formula Categories: Western Herbal Category

* *These categories depend on The Functional Principle of the person and the condition.*

RELEASE THE EXTERIOR	Diaphoretics*
Release Early-Stage Exterior Disorders	Diaphoretics*
Release Exterior Cold	Diaphoretics*
Release Exterior Wind-Heat	Diaphoretics*
Release Exterior Disorders with Head and Neck Symptoms	Diaphoretics*
Release Exterior Disorders with Interior Deficiency	Diaphoretics*
Release Exterior-Interior Excess	Diaphoretics*
CLEAR HEAT	Alteratives, Antacids, Antipyretics, Febrifuges Antibiotics, Antiseptics/Antimicrobials
Clear Heat from Qi Level	Antipyretics, Febrifuges
Clear Heat from Nutritive Level and Cool the Blood	Alteratives, Antipyretics, Febrifuges
Clear Heat and Relieve Toxicity	Antibiotics, Antiseptics/Antimicrobials
Clear Heat form the Organs	Antipyretics
Clear Heat from Deficiency	Non-Available
Relieve Summer heat	Antipyretics
DRAIN DOWNWARD	Cathartics, Cholagogues, Laxatives
Purge Heat Accumulation	Cholagogues
Moisten Intestines and Unblock the Bowels	Laxatives
Warm the Yang and Guide out Accumulation	Non-Available
Drive Out Excess Water	Cathartics
HARMONIZE	Cholagogues, Hepatics, Lithotropics*
Harmonize Gallbladder-Liver Systems	Cholagogues, Hepatics, Lithotropics*
Regulate and Harmonize the Liver-Metabolic-Systems	Hepatics
Harmonize the Stomach-Intestines-Systems	Hepatics
TREAT DRYNESS	Demulcents, Pectorals*
Gently Disperse and Moisten Dryness	Demulcents, Pectorals*
Enrich the Yin and Moisten Dryness	Demulcents, Pectorals*

EXPEL DAMPNESS	Diuretics*
Promote Urination and Leach Out Dampness	Diuretics*
Transform Damp Turbidity	Carminatives + Diuretics*
Clear Damp-Heat	Antipyretics + Diuretics*
Warm and Transform Water and Dampness	Carminatives/Tonics* + Diuretics*
Dispel Wind-Dampness	Analgesics/Anodynes, Antispasmodics + Diuretics
WARM INTERIOR COLD	Digestants, Stimulants
Warm the Channels and Disperse Cold	Carminatives, Digestants
Warm the Middle and Dispel Cold	Carminatives, Digestants
Rescue Devastated Yang	Stimulants
TONIFY (STRENGTHEN)	
Tonify the Qi	Tonics*, Sudorifics*
Tonify Blood	Emmenagogues
Tonify Qi and Blood	Emmenagogues, Tonics
Nourish and Tonify Yin	Emmenagogues, Galactagogues, Nervines, Tonics*, Vulneraries
Warm and Tonify Yang	Stimulants, Tonics*
REGULATE THE QI	Bitters*, Carminatives*, Digestants*, Hepatics*, Sialagogues*
Promote the Movement of Qi	Bitters*, Carminatives*, Digestants, Sialagogues
Direct Rebellious Qi Downward	Carminatives*, Digestants
INVIGORATE THE BLOOD	Emmenagogues*
Invigorate the Blood and Dispel Blood Stasis	Emmenagogues*
Warm the Menses and Dispel Blood Stasis	Emmenagogues*
Invigorate the Blood in the Treatment of Traumatic Injury	Emmenagogues*
STOP BLEEDING	Hemostatics
Clear Heat and Stop Bleeding	Hemostatics*
Tonify and Stop Bleeding	Hemostatics
STABILIZE AND BIND	Astringents
Stabilize the Exterior and the Lungs	Pectorals*
Restrain Leakage from the Intestines	Astringents
Stabilize the Kidney-System	Tonics*
Stabilize the Womb	Emmenagogues*

Notes

Notes

CALM THE SPIRIT (EMOTIONS)	Nervines*, Sedatives*,Soporifics*
Nourish the Heart and Calm the Spirit	Nervines*, Sedatives*, Soporifics*
Sedate and Calm the Spirit	Nervines*, Sedatives*, Soporifics*
EXPEL WIND (AFFECTING MOVEMENT)	Analgesics/Anodynes, Antispasmodics
Release Wind from the Skin and Channels	Analgesics/Anodynes, Antispasmodics
Extinguish Internal Wind	Analgesics/Anodynes, Antispasmodics
OPEN THE ORIFICES (SENSES)	Anticatarrhals*, Carminatives*
Clear Heat and Open Orifices	Anticatarrhals*, Carminatives*
Warm and Open the Orifices	Anticatarrhals*, Carminatives*
Scour Phlegm and Open the Orifices	Anticatarrhals*, Carminatives*
TREAT PHLEGM (TOXIN)	Antiasthmatics, Anticatarrhals, Expectorants, Lithotropics
Dry Dampness and Expel Phlegm	Antiasthmatics, Anticatarrhals, Expectorants, Lithotropics
Clear Heat and Transform Phlegm	Antiasthmatics, Anticatarrhals, Expectorants, Lithotropics
Moisten Dryness and Transform Phlegm	Antiasthmatics, Anticatarrhals, Expectorants, Lithotropics
Transform Phlegm and Dissipate Nodules	Antiasthmatics, Anticatarrhals, Expectorants, Lithotropics
Warm and Transform Cold-Phlegm	Antiasthmatics, Anticatarrhals, Expectorants, Lithotropics
Transform Phlegm and Extinguish Wind	Antiasthmatics, Anticatarrhals, Expectorants, Lithotropics
Induce Vomiting to Discharge Phlegm	Emetics
REDUCE FOOD STAGNATION	Bitters*, Carminatives*, Digestants*
EXPEL PARASITES	Anthelmintics/Parasiticides

Qi Levels of the Body

For correct diagnosis it is essential to know where the disorder lies in the body so the treatment strategies and formulas will target that area.

- **Defensive-Qi**
  Defensive-Qi is the most exterior layer of the body.

- **Qi-Level**
  The Qi-Level is the outermost layer of the interior.

- **Nutritive-Level**
  The Nutritive level is the next deeper level associated with the nutrient carrying Blood-System.

- **Organ-Level**
  The Organ-Level relates to the Qi of each of the Organ-Systems.

Figure–5

QI LEVELS OF THE BODY

Surface

Defensive Qi ______________ Exterior

Qi ______________ Interior

Nutritive ______________

Organ ______________

Bone

Notes

Notes

Treatment Strategies

As noted previously the diagnosis is the foundation of the treatment strategy. The following will describe each category of treatment strategy. Often several strategies can be used simultaneously depending on the situation.

Sweating: Release the Exterior

Strategy: To induce sweating by opening the pores to release the external pathogenic factors with the sweat. In Eastern medicine this is done by assisting the Lung-System that controls the pores. As in the lungs, the pores are open from the inside to the outside of the body. The goal is not the sweating itself but to carry the pathogenic factor out of the body with the sweat. If the person's constitution is weak their energy/Qi may need to be strengthened to help the sweating process. These strategies should not be used long-term as they can weaken the person's system.[6]

Formulas That Release the Exterior Categories:

- **Release Early-Stage Exterior Disorders**
  Response-Pattern: Aversion to wind, fever and chills; used short term.
- **Release Exterior Cold**
  Response-Pattern: Fever and chills (predominant), head and body aches, clear nasal discharge. This presentation can quickly change to Exterior Wind-Heat in which case these formulas should be immediately stopped.
- **Release Exterior Wind-Heat**
  Response-Pattern: Fever, sweating, headache, thirst, sore throat.
- **Release Exterior Disorders with Head and Neck Symptoms**
  Response-Pattern: Wind-heat tends to move upward and will often lodge in the head area.
- **Release Exterior Disorders with Interior Deficiency**
  Response-Pattern: These formulas are used when the person-context is deficient in Qi, Blood, Yin or Yang, and unable to eliminate the pathogenic factor without support.
- **Release Exterior-Interior Excess**
  Response-Pattern: These formulas are used when the pathogenic factor is still present in the exterior but is also affecting the interior, such as a flu with heat rashes, nosebleeds, or diarrhea.

Formulas That Clear Heat

Strategy: To clear heat (not in the exterior) and drain fire and toxicity. This method is used for various causes of interior and/or organ-system excess heat with acute presentations.[7]

The herbs in these formulas are cold in their Functional Principle and can injure the Stomach and Metabolic-Systems and should be discontinued as soon as the excess heat is resolved.

Clear Heat Formula Categories:

- **Clear Heat from Qi-Level**
  Response-Pattern: High fever, profuse sweating, irritability, thirst.
- **Clear Heat from the Nutritive Level and Cool the Blood**
  Response-Pattern: Fever that gets worse at night, irritability, insomnia, rashes, bleeding, Blood stasis.
- **Clear Heat and Relieve Toxicity**
  Response-Pattern: Excess heat and toxin with fever, irritability, nausea or vomiting, nosebleed, rashes, sores, upper body.
- **Clear Heat from the Organs**
  Response-Pattern: Where the presentation is in an organ-system.
- **Clear Heat from Deficiency (and Enrich Yin Fluids)**
  Response-Pattern: Excess heat where the body is depleted or deficient in Essential Fluids.
- **Relieve Summerheat**
  Response-Pattern: Usually in late summer, high fever and profuse sweating, injured Qi and Fluids, thirst, irritability.

Formulas That Drain Downward

Strategy: To induce bowel movements (laxative) to cleanse and remove accumulation in the Intestinal-System. These can be harsh formulas and should not be used long-term as they can injure the Qi-energy of the Metabolic-System.

Constipation can be caused by the pathogenic influences of dryness, heat, or cold leading to accumulation, or simply the accumulation and stagnation of water or blood.[8]

Drain Downward Formula Categories:

- **Purge Heat Accumulation**
  Response-Pattern: Interior excess with fever, abdominal pain increasing with pressure, constipation, yellow tongue coat.
- **Moisten the Intestines and Unblock the Bowels**
  Response-Pattern: Intestinal dryness creating constipation.
- **Warm the Yang and Guide Out Accumulation**
  Response-Pattern: Cold excess with constipation, abdominal fullness or pain that responds to warmth.[9]
- **Drive Out Excess Water**
  Response-Pattern: Accumulation of water or fluids obstructing Qi-energy flow in the abdomen causing constipation.

Formulas That Harmonize

Strategy: To harmonize and/or regulate the functions of organs or tissues. This strategy is used when two or more Systems are not working together harmoniously. Harmonizing involves disorders that are considered partly exterior and partly interior such as, melancholia,

Notes

Notes

painful menstruation, and/or distention of the abdomen. The organ-systems involved are usually the Liver, Metabolic, Gallbladder, Stomach, and Intestines. These are the most frequently used formulas in a clinic.

The presentation can involve heat and cold separately or simultaneously.

Harmonizing Formula Categories:

- **Harmonize the Liver and Gallbladder-System (also known as Lesser-Yang-Stage)**
  Response-Pattern: Dry throat, bitter taste, fullness in the upper abdomen, alternating fever and chills.
- **Harmonize the Liver and Metabolic-Systems**
  Response-Pattern: Abdominal pain or distention, poor appetite, diarrhea, suppressed anger and/or frustration.
- **Harmonize the Stomach and Intestinal-Systems**
  Response-Pattern: Abdominal distention and/or pain, nausea, vomiting, borborygmus, diarrhea.

Formulas That Treat Dryness

Strategy: To disperse and moisten internal dryness using herbs to enrich the Yin or moisten.

External dryness disorders can vary according to the climate, the time of year and the use of indoor heating and air conditioning that can dry and injure the Lung-System.

Internal dryness can result from the depletion of Fluids from excessive sweating, vomiting, diarrhea, to eating overly spicy-hot foods.

The herbs in these formulas are mostly rich and heavy, which can easily overwhelm the Metabolic-System and may need to be modified for each person.

Treat Dryness Formula Categories:

- **Gently Disperse and Moisten Dryness**
  Response-Pattern: Cough with sparse mucus. Cool-dryness presents with chills, headache, dry mouth and throat. Warm dryness presents with fever, headache, thirst, and irritability.[10]
- **Enrich the Yin and Moisten Dryness**
  Response-Pattern: Cough with little mucus, nausea, vomiting, dry mouth, thirst, constipation.

Formulas That Expel Dampness

Dampness is most often correlated with poor food choices, irregular eating habits, excessive mental work, and/or living in a damp climate. The Metabolic-System is affected, which then cannot properly transform food and Fluids. The results can be poor digestion, nausea, vomiting, diarrhea, painful urination, edema of the lower body, or pain in the joints. Dampness can also be attributed to the Kidney-System which can cause difficulty with urination, and edema of the lower body.

The herbs in these formulas are mostly acrid, aromatic and warm which can injure the Essential Fluids.

Notes

Expel Dampness Formula Categories:

- **Promote Urination and Leach Out Dampness**
  Response-Pattern: Edema, urinary difficulty or pain.
- **Transform Damp Turbidity (Viscosity)**
  Response-Pattern: Abdominal distention, belching, acid regurgitation, vomiting, diarrhea, poor appetite, tiredness. The aromatic herbs in these formulas disperse the viscous nature of the dampness.
- **Clear Damp-Heat**
  Response-Pattern: Sensations of heat that increase in the afternoon, feelings of heaviness, painful urination, burning sensations in the lower body, yellow thick tongue coating.
- **Warm and Transform Water and Dampness**
  Response-Pattern: Difficult or scanty urination, poor appetite, or lower body edema.
- **Dispel Wind-Dampness**
  Response-Pattern: Numbness and pain in the joints due to dampness obstructing the Qi-energy flow.

Formulas That Warm Interior Cold

Strategy: To warm and disperse cold from the interior and channels, and restore the normal flow of Qi-energy which has been restricted due to the contracting nature of cold.[11] These formulas are different from those that strengthen the Yang which are more tonifying in nature.

The herbs in these formulas are hot and drying in Functional Principles and can injure the Essential Fluids if used inappropriately.

Warm Interior Cold Formula Categories:

- **Warm the Channels and Disperse Cold**
  Response-Pattern: Coldness, pale tongue, Blood deficiency, pain.
- **Warm the Middle and Dispel Cold**
  Response-Pattern: Cold in the Metabolic-System causing abdominal distention and pain, tiredness, poor appetite, feelings of coldness, white tongue coat.
- **Rescue Devastated Yang**
  Response-Pattern: Exhaustion and collapse of Qi-energy with coldness and aversion to cold, sweating, shortness of breath.

Tonifying Formulas

Strategy: To strengthen by nourishing, supplementing, and/or replenishing weak or deficient systems or tissues of the body such as deficient Qi-energy, Blood, Yin, Yang, or organ-systems.[12] These formulas are rich and heavy and should be used only in cases of true deficiency and may need to be modified to assist the Metabolic-System in digesting them.

Notes

Tonifying Formula Categories:

- **Tonify the Qi**
  Response-Pattern: These formulas are used to strengthen the Metabolic and Lung-Systems. There may be symptoms of fatigue and tiredness which get worse with activity and improves with rest.
- **Tonify the Blood**
  Response-Pattern: Dizziness, pale tongue and lips, dry lips and nails, palpitations, insomnia, menstrual problems with scanty flow.
- **Tonify Qi and Blood**
  Response-Pattern: Light-headed, palpitations, tiredness, pale tongue and complexion.
- **Nourish and Tonify the Yin**
  Response-Pattern: Depleted Essential Fluids (deficient Yin) usually involving the Liver and Kidney-Systems with sore and weak lower back, irritability, evening rise in heat, night sweats, insomnia, red tongue with little to no coating. These formulas are rich and heavy and used with caution if the Metabolic-System is weak.
- **Warm and Tonify the Yang**
  Response-Pattern: Deficiency with coldness, sore or weak lower back and legs, tiredness, pale tongue, frequent and excessive urination, morning diarrhea, watery vaginal discharge, impotence.

Formulas That Regulate the Qi

Strategy: To reestablish the flow of Qi-energy especially of the Liver and Metabolic-Systems that present with pain and abdominal distention due to emotional upset and irregular eating habits. It is important to determine which organ-system is involved and whether it is hot or cold, and excess or deficient in nature.

The herbs in these formulas are generally bitter or acrid and warming or drying in Functional Principles.

Regulate the Qi Formula Categories:

- **Promote the Movement of Qi**
  Response-Pattern: Pain either in the chest or abdominal area, irregular menses. These formulas work with the Liver and Metabolic-Systems.
- **Direct Rebellious (Reversed) Qi Downward**
  Response-Pattern: Coughing, wheezing, vomiting, belching involving the Lung or Stomach-Systems where the Qi-energy is moving opposite to the normal flow.

Formulas that Invigorate the Blood

Strategy: To treat blockage or reduced blood flow due to poor or blocked Qi-energy, cold constricting, or heat drying (thickening) the Blood.

These formulas should not be used in pregnancy or in people with deficiencies such as Blood deficiency.

Notes

Formulas That Invigorate the Blood Categories:

- **Invigorate the Blood and Dispel Blood Stasis**
  Response-Pattern: Static Blood with deep severe pain, immobile masses, abscesses, purple lips or tongue.
- **Warm the Menses and Dispel Blood Stasis**
  Response-Pattern: Due to cold there may be delayed menstruation, dark menstrual blood with clots, pale purple tongue.
- **Invigorate the Blood in the Treatment of Traumatic Injury**
  Response-Pattern: To treat swelling and pain from traumatic injuries.

Formulas that Stop Bleeding

Strategy: To stop excessive bleeding from various pathological factors such as excess heat, Blood or Qi deficiency.

Stop Bleeding Formula Categories:

- **Clear Heat and Stop Bleeding**
  Response-Pattern: Rashes, nosebleeds, coughing of blood, blood in the urine or stool due to excess heat.
- **Tonify and Stop Bleeding**
  Response-Pattern: Bleeding due to deficiency especially of the Metabolic-System.

Formulas that Stabilize and Bind

Strategy: To stop the leakage of fluids such as blood, urine, stool, sweat, vaginal discharge. The herbs in these formulas are astringent.

Stabilize and Bind Formula Categories:

- **Stabilize the Exterior and the Lungs**
  Response-Pattern: Spontaneous sweating, pale complexion, shortness of breath, night sweats, pale tongue.
- **Restrain Leakage from the Intestines**
  Response-Pattern: Excessive diarrhea, incontinence of stools, weakness, tiredness, poor appetite, pale tongue.
- **Stabilize the Kidneys**
  Response-Pattern: Bladder incontinence, weak and sore lower back, tinnitus, forgetfulness, pale tongue with white coating.
- **Stabilize the Womb**
  Response-Pattern: Uterine bleeding and vaginal discharge that is chronic, palpitations, shortness of breath, weak and sore lower back, pale complexion, pale tongue.

Notes

Formulas that Calm the Spirit (Emotions)

Strategy: To calm anxiety and agitation by nourishing the Blood and Yin to quiet the emotions.

Calm the Spirit Formula Categories:

- **Nourish the Heart and Calm the Spirit**
  Response-Pattern: Palpitations, irritability, insomnia due to deficiency of Blood and Yin of the Heart-System.
- **Sedate and Calm the Spirit**
  Response-Pattern: Anxiety or phobias, restlessness, erratic emotional outbursts.

Formulas that Expel Wind (Affects Movement)

Strategy: To treat wind causing itching, numbness of the skin, spasms, stiff or painful joints.

The herbs in these formulas are warming and drying in nature and can injure the Essential Fluids.

Expel Wind Formula Categories:

- **Release Wind from the Skin and Channels**
  Response-Pattern: Rashes, itching, dizziness, numbness, stiff movement, joint pain.
- **Extinguish Internal Wind**
  Response-Pattern: headaches, dizziness, blurred vision, tinnitus, palpitations with anxiety, muscle twitches, spasms, tremors or asymmetry of the face.

Formulas that Open the Orifices (Senses)

Strategy: To improve the senses by unblocking the Qi-energy.

The presentation can be either hot or cold, excess or deficient. The strong dispersing action of these herbs can injure the Qi.

Open the Orifices Formula Categories:

- **Clear Heat and Open the Orifices**
  Response-Pattern: high fever, irritability, restlessness, red face, heavy breathing, spasms, convulsions, yellow tongue coat.
- **Warm and Open the Orifices**
  Response-Pattern: Clenching of the jaw, cold body, white tongue coat.
- **Scour Phlegm and Open the Orifices**
  Response-Pattern: Dull senses, raspy sound in throat, greasy looking tongue coat.

Formulas that Treat Phlegm (Toxin)

Notes

Strategy: To strengthen the Metabolic-System (the source of dampness and phlegm), dry dampness, expel phlegm. Phlegm is a sticky, thick "substance" that can block the Qi-energy, channels, sensory organs, and functions.

The presentation can be hot or cold in Functional Principle.

Treat Phlegm Formula Categories:

- **Dry Dampness and Expel Phlegm**
  Response-Pattern: Excessive clear or white easily expelled mucus, nausea, weak extremities, headache, palpitations, anxiety.
- **Clear Heat and Transform Phlegm**
  Response-Pattern: Coughing of thick, yellow, sticky mucus that is difficult to expel, red face, yellow tongue coat.
- **Moisten Dryness and Transform Phlegm**
  Response-Pattern: Difficult to expel thick, sticky mucus due to dryness.
- **Transform Phlegm and Dissipate Nodules**
  Response-Pattern: Subcutaneous nodules, cysts.
- **Warm and Transform Cold-Phlegm**
  Response-Pattern: Coughing of thin white mucus, coldness, white, slippery tongue coat.
- **Transform Phlegm and Extinguish Wind**
  Response-Pattern: Aversion to wind, coughing of excess mucus, dizziness, headache, seizures.
- **Induce Vomiting to Discharge Phlegm**
  Response-Pattern: Excess phlegm, poisoning, food accumulation.

Formulas that Reduce Food Stagnation

Strategy: To disperse stagnation and accumulation of food in the digestive system with abdominal distention and bloating, aversion to food, belching with a bad odor.

The herbs in these formulas are strongly dispersing and can therefore injure the Qi.

Formulas that Expel Parasites

Strategy: To expel parasites from the digestive tract.

Notes

Chapter 13:

The Physic-Systems of Herbal Medicine

'Perversity of mind' is the ultimate cause of every disease.
—Robert Svoboda, Ayurvedic Physician[1]

In this chapter, the classifications of Western herbal medicine and the systems of Ayurveda and Chinese Medicine will be integrated using The Five Phases and The Six Tastes and as discussed in Chapters 5 and 6. The purpose is to provide a consistent systems-based framework to use Western herbs more effectively and for the Western herbalist or medical doctor to become familiar with a descriptive system-based terminology that is not symptomatic in its approach.

Terminology of Herbal Medicine

Part of the confusion in the field of herbal medicine comes from the lack of consistent terminology to describe how herbs act on the body. Western herbal medicine lacks a comprehensive foundation in principles and strategies to accurately describe the actions of the herbs other than symptomatically; Eastern medicine uses terminology that is unfamiliar to the Western mind.

In the following, when discussing Phases, Tastes, and Functional Principles, the general or most used Functional Principles of the herbs are cited. For example, in the Western category of Antacids, the herbs used are always cooling in Functional Principle since an acid condition is always one of heat or inflammation. However, in the category of Anti-Asthmatics, the Functional Principle of the herbs used could be cool or warm depending on The Functional Principles of the condition being treated.

For example, if the condition is one of heat and inflammation, the herbs used would be cooling and moistening. If the condition were cold and wet the herbs used would be warming and drying. Western herbal medicine does not differentiate conditions into these presentations.

Notes

Table–13-1

THE EIGHT PROPERTIES OF THE SIX TASTES

Context—Process—Experience

	SWEET	SOUR	SALTY	PUNGENT	BITTER	ASTRINGENT
Phases	*Water Earth*	*Fire Earth*	*Fire Water*	*Air Fire*	*Space Air*	*Space Earth*
COOLING	✕				✕	✕
HEATING		✕	✕	✕		
DRYING		✕		✕	✕	✕
MOISTENING	✕	✕	✕			
UPWARD				✕	✕	✕
DOWNWARD	✕	✕	✕			
INWARD		✕				✕
OUTWARD				✕	✕	

This ambiguity can be cleared up by dividing herbs into categories according to their Tastes, and then, their proportionate Phases. Therefore, the Functional Principle will be noted "Varies" to denote that The Functional Principles of the herbs used vary according to what is needed to counteract the Functional Principle of the condition.

In addition to the Western herbal classifications, the Western herbal medicine uses of each category are noted. Comments are then noted to expand on those uses from an Eastern medicine perspective.

The Western herbal examples are not a complete listing of all the herbs in a category. Generally, as mentioned previously, herbs should be used as formulations not singularly to avoid adverse effects.

Also noted where possible, is what chemical constituents are generally present in each category, or noted "varies" if it contains many different chemical constituents.

To determine the dominant Phases, Tastes, and Functional Principles of each of the Western therapeutics, the *Chinese Herbal Medicine Materia Medica* and *Planetary Herbology* were used where the Taste and Functional Principle is listed for each herb. (See Chapter 8.)

Notes

If an herb was listed as cool, then Air is predominant. If it was listed as cold, then Space is predominant. Each Phase and Taste is listed in order of predominance.

Note: To denote pathological conditions in the body, terms such as Heat, Cold, Wet, Damp, Dry, Wind, will be capitalized.

Therapeutics of Western Herbs Integrated with the Systems of Ayurveda and Chinese Medicine

Alteratives

Western: These herbs are termed as blood purifiers and are used to "detoxify" the blood.
Comments: Alterative herbs are used to treat inflammations, and skin conditions caused by Heat (toxins) in the Blood-System such as boils, acne, rashes. These Heat clearing herbs will treat conditions caused by excess Heat in the Blood such as nosebleed, vomiting, spitting or coughing of blood, and blood in the stool or urine caused by high fevers. These conditions create inflammation in the organs that further increase the internal Heat causing increased permeability of the capillaries and therefore bleeding.[2]
Western Herbal Examples:

- Burdock, root *Arctium lappa*
- Dandelion, root, *Taraxacum officinale*
- Honeysuckle, flower, *Lonicera japonica*
- Oregon Grape, root, *Mahonia repens*
- Red Clover, flower, *Trifolium pratense*
- Sarsaparilla, root, *Smilax officinalis*

Chemical Constituents: Bitter compounds
Phases: Space, Air, Water, Earth
Taste: Bitter, Sweet
Functional Principle: Cold
Chinese Medicine: Herbs that Clear Heat and Cool the Blood
Ayurveda: Herbs that reduce Pitta

Analgesics/Anodynes

Western: These are used to reduce pain and so have a calming effect on the nervous system; some can be antispasmodic (reduces Wind or Vata) and reduce cramping.
Comments: The calming effect of these herbs is due to their ability to remove a stimulus (Pathogenic Factor) that is aggravating the nervous system such as Wind, Cold or Dryness. (See Chapter 5.) Dryness, for example, can create Heat (inflammation) and therefore internal Wind-Heat and pain. Cold creates stagnation, which then causes pain.
Western Herbal Examples:

- Black Haw, bark, *Viburnum prunifolium*
- California Poppy, aerial parts, *Eschscholzia californica*
- Cramp Bark, bark, *Viburnum opulis*

- Jamaican Dogwood, bark, *Piscidia piscipula*
- Kava, root, *Piper methysticum*

Chemical Constituents: varies
Phases: Air, Water, Earth, Fire
Taste: Salty, Acrid
Functional Principle: Varies
Chincse Medicine: Herbs that Extinguish Wind and Stop Tremors
Ayurveda: Herbs that reduce Vata

Notes

Antacids

Western: These herbs are used to neutralize excess acids in the stomach and intestines that create inflammation or toxic conditions.
Comments: These herbs help with heartburn (reflux), hiatal hernia, and ulcers caused by excess Heat usually of the Liver-System whose warming Functional Principle moves upward to disturb the Stomach. If this condition continues over time the Stomach-moisture (Yin) will be depleted leading to ulcers. Consistent consumption of hot-spicy foods will also cause depletion of Stomach-moisture.
Western Herbal Examples:

- Dandelion, leaf and root, *Taraxacum officinale*
- Irish Moss, whole plant, *Chondrus crispus*
- Psyllium, seed, *Plantago psyllium*
- Slippery Elm, inner bark, *Ulmus fulva*

Chemical Constituents: Bitter compounds
Phases: Space, Air, Water, Earth
Taste: Bitter, Sweet
Functional Principle: Cold
Chinese Medicine: Herbs that Drain Fire
Ayurveda: Herbs that reduce Pitta and increase Kapha

Anthelmintics/Parasiticides

Western: These are used to help eliminate parasites, yeast, and fungus.
Comments: Because of their dispersing effect (Air and Space Phases) these herbs can be draining to the body and should not be used long-term without being modified by other herbs that offset their draining properties.
The Functional Principle varies because most parasitical conditions can be eliminated by Cold herbs. Yeast and fungus will more often respond to more warming (Fire Phase) herbs.
Western Herbal Examples:

- Betel Nut, seeds, *Areca catechu*
- Garlic, bulb, *Allium sativa*
- Male Fern, rhizome, *Dryopteris filix-mas*
- Pink Root, root, *Spigelia marilandica*
- Pomegranate, peel of fruit, bark, *Punica granatum*
- Pumpkin, seed, husk, *Curcubita maxima*

Notes

Chemical Constituents: Varies
Phases: Air, Space, Earth, Fire
Taste: Bitter, Acrid
Functional Principle: Varies
Chinese Medicine: Herbs that Expel Parasites
Ayurveda: Herbs that reduce Pitta and Kapha

Antiasthmatics

Western: Used to help relieve the symptoms of asthma by either/or moistening, dilating the bronchioles, and breaking up mucus.
Comments: The cause of Lung conditions vary greatly. Some Lung conditions can be Hot (inflammation); some can be simply Dry, like a dry cough after a cold or flu or a more serious condition of consumption (Dry and Hot); some can be Hot and Wet (excess mucous) or Cold and Wet; some can be simply Wet. The correct diagnosis is crucial to using the right herbs.
Western Herbal Examples:

- Coltsfoot, leaf, flower, *Tussilago farfara*
- Comfrey, leaf and root, *Symphytum officinale*
- Elecampane, root, *Inula japonica*
- Lobelia, leaf, flower, seeds, *Lobelia inflata*
- Mullein, leaf, flower, root, *Verbascum thapsus*
- Pleurisy Root, root, *Asclepias tuberosa*
- Yerba Santa, leaf, *Erodictyon spp.*

Chemical Constituents: Varies
Phases: Air, Earth, Space, Fire, Water
Taste: Bitter, Acrid, Sweet
Functional Principle: Varies
Chinese Medicine: Herbs that Relieve Coughing and Wheezing
Ayurveda: Herbs that reduce Kapha or Vata

Antibiotics

Western: Meaning "anti-life," these herbs are said to have "germ killing abilities" and can stimulate the body's defense systems against infectious conditions. These are some of the coldest herbs in any material medica. These herbs ". . . do not destroy the bacteria but prevent them from multiplying, so that mutations cannot occur and strains of bacteria resistant to the medication are unlikely to develop."[3] The immune system can then more easily overcome the infection.
Comments: Western herbalism has many wonderful herbs in this category that are highly effective and useful.
Western Herbal Examples:

- Andrographitis, aerial parts, *Andrographis paniculata*
- Begonia, aerial parts, *Begonia spp.*
- Blue Flag, rhizome, *Iris versicolor*

- Chaparral, leaf, *Larrea tridentata*
- Chrysanthemum, flower, *Chrysanthemum indicum*
- Dandelion, root, leaf, *Taraxacum officinale*
- Echinacea, root, *Echinacea spp.*
- Forsythia, fruit, *Forsythia suspensa*
- Goldenseal, root, *Hydrastis canadensis*
- Honeysuckle, flower, *Lonicera japonica*
- Pulsatilla, root, *Pulsatilla chinensis*
- Purslane, leaf, *Portulaca oleracea*
- Usnea, whole plant, *Usnea spp.*
- Violet, flower, rhizome, *Viola odorata*

Chemical Constituents: Bitter compounds
Phases: Space, Air
Taste: Bitter
Functional Principle: Cold
Chinese Medicine: Herbs that Clear Heat and Relieve Toxicity
Ayurveda: Herbs that reduce Pitta

Notes

Anticatarrhals

Western: Used to eliminate and prevent excessive catarrhal (mucus) buildup in the Lung-System or other parts of the body.
Comments: The pattern of excessive mucus and Phlegm (pathogenic mucus) is poor digestion. Mucus is sent up to the Lungs (includes the sinuses) where it can be stored. However, Phlegm can be present anywhere in the body and contributes to conditions such as goiter and cysts (often combined with Fire). Phlegm can also clog the channels of the body and create stroke (when combined with Wind) and other mental disorders. Because the pattern of the condition can be one of Cold or Heat, the Functional Principle varies.
Western Herbal Examples:
Cooling:

- Bamboo, sap, shavings, *Bambusa breviflora*
- Chickweed, aerial parts, *Stellaria dichotoma*
- Clam, shell, *Cyclinae sinensis*
- Horehound, leaf, *Marrubium vulgare*
- Kelp, *Laminaria japonica*
- Pumice
- Sargassum, *Sargassum pallidum*

Warming:

- Balloon Flower, root, *Platycodon grandiflorum*
- Bloodroot, root, *Sanguinaria canadensis*
- Elecampane, root, *Inula japonica*
- Eucalyptus, leaf, *Eucalyptus globulus*
- Grindelia, leaf and flower, *Grindelia spp.*
- Mustard, seed, *Brassica alba*

Notes

- Thyme, leaf and flower, *Thymus vulgaris*
- Yerba Santa, leaf, *Eriodictyon spp.*

Chemical Constituents: Varies
Phases: Space, Air, Water, Earth, Fire
Taste: Bitter, Sweet, Pungent
Functional Principle: Varies
Chinese Medicine: Herbs that Cool/Warm Transform Phlegm-Cold/Heat
Ayurveda: Herbs that reduce Kapha, Pitta

Antipyretics

Western: Used to reduce fevers.
Comments: These are the coldest herbs in any materia medica and are often combined with Herbs that Clear Heat and Relieve Toxicity. Additional herbs should be added to protect the Stomach and Metabolic-Systems.
Western Herbal/Mineral Examples:

- Calcium, mineral
- Celosia, seed, *Celosia argentea*
- Gardenia, fruit, *Gardenia jasminoides*
- Gypsum, mineral
- Self-Heal, flowering part, *Prunella vulgaris*
- Violet, whole plant, *Viola odorata*

Chemical Constituents: Mostly bitter compounds
Phases: Space, Air, Water, Earth
Taste: Bitter, Sweet
Functional Principle: Cold
Chinese Medicine: Herbs that Drain Fire
Ayurveda: Herbs that reduce Pitta

Antiseptics/Anti-Microbial

See Antibiotics
Western: Used to help prevent the growth of bacteria. See Antibiotics.
Comments: Theses herbs are very Cold and should be combined with herbs that protect the Stomach and Metabolic-Systems.
Western Herbal Examples:

- Andrographitis, aerial parts, *Andrographis paniculata*
- Begonia, aerial parts, *Begonia spp.*
- Blue Flag, rhizome, *Iris versicolor*
- Chaparral, leaf, *Larrea tridentata*
- Chrysanthemum, flower, *Chrysanthemum indicum*
- Dandelion, root, *Taraxacum officinale*
- Echinacea, root, *Echinacea spp.*
- Forsythia, fruit, *Forsythia suspensa*
- Goldenseal, root, *Hydrastis canadensis*

- Honeysuckle, root, *Lonicera japonica*
- Pulsatilla, root, *Pulsatilla chinensis*
- Purslane, aerial parts, *Portulaca oleracea*
- Usnea, whole plant, *Usnea spp.*
- Violet, whole plant, *Viola odorata*

Chemical Constituents: bitter compounds
Phases: Space, Air
Taste: Bitter
Functional Principle: Cold
Chinese Medicine: Herbs that Clear Heat and Relieve Toxicity
Ayurveda: Herbs that reduce Pitta

Notes

Anti-Spasmodics

Western: Used to prevent or ease cramps and muscle spasms in the body.
Comments: Cramps and spasms occur due to pathogenic Wind in the body which these herbs help to reduce. The causes of pathogenic Wind vary and determines which herbs will be used. See Analgesics/Anodynes.
Western Herbal Examples:

- Abalone, shell, *Haliotis diversicolor*
- Black Haw, bark, *Viburnum prunifolium*
- Caltrop, fruit, *Tribulus terrestris*
- Cramp Bark, bark, *Viburnum opulis*
- Gastrodia, rhizome, *Gastrodia elata*
- Lobelia, leaf, flower, seed, *Lobelia inflata*
- Uncaria, stem and thorn, *Uncaria sinensis*

Chemical Constituents: Varies
Phases: Fire, Water, Earth, Air
Taste: Salty, Acrid
Functional Principle: Varies
Chinese Medicine: Substances that Extinguish Wind and Stop Tremors
Ayurveda: Herbs that reduce Vata

Astringents

Western: Used to constrict tissues thereby reducing discharge and secretions.
Comments: These herbs have diverse functions such as to stop sweating, diarrhea, excessive urination or bleeding. The pattern of these conditions is most often some form of deficiency which should be addressed after the person and the condition is stabilized.
Western Herbal Examples:

- Amaranth, aerial parts, *Amaranthus spp.*
- Bistort, root, *Bistorta officinalis*
- Blackberry, leaves, root bark, *Rubus spp.*
- Cranesbill, root, *Geranium spp.*
- Ephedra, root, *Ephedra spp.*

Notes

- Eyebright, aerial parts, *Euphrasia officinalis*
- Gingko, seed, *Ginkgo biloba*
- Horse Chestnut, seed and bark, *Aesculus hippocastanum*
- Lady's Mantle, aerial parts, *Alchemilla vulgaris*
- Nettles, leaf, *Urtica dioica*
- Nutmeg, seed, *Myristica fragrans*
- Oak, bark, acorn, *Quercus spp.*
- Pomegranate, peel of fruit, *Punica granatum*
- Raspberry, fruit, *Rubus chingii*
- Rosehip, fruit, *Rosa rugosa*
- Schisandra, fruit, *Schisandra sinensis*
- Sumac, root bark, berry, *Rhus glabra*
- Witch Hazel, leaf, bark, *Hamemelis virginiana*
- Yerba Mansa, root, leaf, *Anemopsis californica*

Chemical Constituents: Tannins
Phases: Air, Earth
Taste: Astringent
Functional Principle: Cool
Chinese Medicine: Herbs that Stabilize and Bind
Ayurveda: Herbs that reduce Kapha

Bitters

Western: Used to stimulate the digestive system.
Comments: Bitters are Cold herbs and therefore would be used in conditions of stagnation causing Heat (inflammation). They would not be used in every case of digestive problems as many digestive conditions could be due to Cold conditions which these herbs would aggravate.
Western Herbal Examples:

- Gentian, root, *Gentiana lutea*
- Goldenseal, root, *Hydrastis canadensis*
- Wormwood, aerial parts, *Artemisia annua*

Chemical Constituents: Bitter compounds
Phases: Air, Space, Earth, Fire
Taste: Bitter
Functional Principle: Cold
Chinese Medicine: Herbs that Regulate Qi
Ayurveda: Herbs that reduce Pitta

Carminatives

Western: Used to stimulate the digestive system these herbs help to release gas and griping in the bowels.
Comments: These are warming and drying herbs to counter Dampness and Cold obstructing the Metabolic-System that could cause griping.

Western Herbal Examples:

- Caraway, seed, *Carum carvi*
- Cardamom, fruit, *Amomum villosum*
- Chive, bulb, *Allium macrostemon*
- Citrus, peel of fruit, *Citrus reticulata*
- Cumin, seed, *Cuminum cyminum*
- Cyperus, rhizome, *Cyperus rotundus*
- Galangal, rhizome, *Alpinia officinarum*
- Magnolia, bark, *Magnolia officinalis*
- Patchouli, aerial parts, *Agastache rugosa*
- Rose, flower, *Rosa rugosa*
- Sandalwood, heartwood, *Santalum album*
- Tangerine, peel of fruit, *Citri reticulata*

Chemical Constituents: Volatile oils
Phases: Air, Fire
Taste: Pungent
Functional Principle: Warm
Chinese Medicine: Aromatic Herbs That Transform Dampness; Herbs that Regulate the Qi
Ayurveda: Herbs that reduce Vata and Kapha

Notes

Cathartics

Western: Used as a purgative; stimulates peristalsis and can produce irritation and griping.
Comments: These herbs work on constipation due to accumulation of Heat in the intestinal tract and are considered harsh. See also Laxatives and Purgatives.
Western Herbal Examples:

- Elder, bark, *Sambucus canadensis*
- Mandrake, rhizome, *Mandragora spp.*
- Morning Glory, seed, *Ipomoea spp.*
- Poke Root, root, *Phytolacca acinosa.*
- Scotch Broom, flower, *Cytisus scoparius*

Chemical Constituents: Bitter compounds
Phases: Space, Air
Taste: Bitter
Functional Principle: Cold
Chinese Medicine: Downward Draining Herbs: Harsh Expellants
Ayurveda: Herbs that reduce Pitta

Cholagogues

Western: Used to promote the flow of bile to purge the colon.
Comments: These Cold herbs are used for constipation due to Heat accumulation in the Liver and Gallbladder-Systems caused by Qi stagnation.
Western Herbal Examples:

- Aloe, leaf, *Aloe vera*

Notes

- Barberry, root, *Berberis vulgaris*
- Dandelion, root, *Taraxacum officinale*
- Gentian, root, *Gentiana lutea*
- Goldenseal, root, *Hydrastis canadensis*
- Rhubarb, root, *Rheum palmatum*

Chemical Constituents: Bitter compounds
Phases: Space, Air
Taste: Bitter
Functional Principle: Cold
Chinese Medicine: Herbs That Clear Heat; Downward Draining Herbs: Purgatives
Ayurveda: Herbs that reduce Pitta

Demulcents

Western: Rich in mucilage, used to soothe and heal irritated and inflamed tissue.
Comments: These herbs are moistening and therefore, Cooling and nourishing.
Western Herbal Examples:

- Aloe, leaf, *Aloe vera*
- Chia, seed, *Salvia hispanica*
- Chickweed, aerial parts, *Stellaria media*
- Comfrey, leaf, root, *Symphytum officinale*
- Fenugreek, seed, *Trigonella foenum-graecum*
- Flax, seed, *Linum usitatissimum*
- Irish Moss, whole plant, *Chondrus crispus*
- Licorice, root, *Glycyrrhiza glabra*
- Marshmallow, root, *Althea officinalis*
- Mullein, flower, leaf, root, *Verbascum thapsus*
- Oats, seed, *Avena sativa*
- Psyllium, seed, *Plantago psyllium*
- Slippery Elm, inner bark, *Ulmus fulva*

Chemical Constituents: Polysaccharides
Phases: Water, Earth, Air, Space
Taste: Sweet, Bitter
Functional Principle: Cool
Chinese Medicine: Herbs that Tonify Yin
Ayurveda: Herbs that increase Kapha, reduce Vata, Pitta

Diaphoretics

Western: Helps to induce sweating. Diaphoretics are to be taken hot; when given cool they tend to act as diuretics.
Comments: These herbs are used to dislodge a pathogenic factor that has not yet penetrated the body such as Wind-Heat, Wind-Cold, or Wind-Damp which are the first symptoms of a cold or flu such as chills, fever, headache, muscle aches, and some rashes. By opening the pores, sweating occurs which expels the pathogen. The Functional Principle

varies depending on whether the Functional Principle of the condition is one of Heat or Cold. Using the wrong herbs (Functional Principle) at the wrong time can make the condition worse.

Western Herbal Examples:

Warming:

- Basil, aerial parts, *Ocimum basilicum*
- Catnip, leaf, *Nepeta cataria*
- Cinnamon, twig, *Cinnamon cassia*
- Costmary, leaf, *Tanacetum balsamita*
- Ephedra, aerial parts, *Ephedra spp.*
- Ginger, rhizome, *Zingiberis officinalis*
- Hyssop, aerial parts, *Hyssopus officinalis*
- Lovage, root, *Ligusticum levisticum*
- Magnolia, flower, *Magnolia officinalis*
- Marjoram, aerial parts, *Origanum majorana*
- Oregano, aerial parts, *Origanum vulgare*
- Osha, root, *Ligusticum porteri*
- Sage, leaf, *Salvia officinalis*
- Savory, aerial parts, *Satureja hortensis*
- Scallion, bulb, *Allium fistulosum*
- Wild Ginger, whole plant, *Asarum canadense*
- Yerba Buena, aerial parts, *Satureja douglasii*

Cooling:

- Elder, flower, *Sambucus nigra*
- Peppermint, leaves, *Mentha piperita*
- Yarrow, flower, leaf, *Achillea millefolium*

Chemical Constituents: Polysaccharides
Phases: Air, Fire, Water, Earth
Taste: Acrid, Bitter, Sweet
Functional Principle: Varies
Chinese Medicine: Warm/Cool Acrid Herbs that Release the Exterior
Ayurveda: Herbs that reduce Pitta and Vata

Digestants

Western: Used to help digest food.
Comments: Herbs that warm and relieve pathological Cold as opposed to tonifying or strengthening Yang—and tend to be Hot and Dry in nature.[4] They should be used in small amounts with caution so as not to imbalance the system.

Western Herbal Examples:

- Capsicum, fruit, *Capsicum frutescens*
- Chive, bulb, *Allium macrostemon*
- Cinnamon, bark, *Cinnamon cassia*
- Clove, flower bud, *Caryophyllus aromaticus*
- Fennel, fruit, *Foeniculum vulgare*

Notes

Notes

- Ginger, rhizome, *Zingiberis officinalis*
- Pepper, fruit, *Piper nigrum*
- Rose, flower, *Rosa rugosa*
- Sandalwood, heartwood, *Santalum album*
- Tangerine, peel of fruit, *Citri reticulata*

Chemical Constituents: Varies
Phases: Fire
Taste: Pungent
Functional Principle: Warm, Hot
Chinese Medicine: Herbs that Regulate the Qi, or Warm the Interior and Dispel Cold
Ayurveda: Herbs that reduce Vata and Kapha and increase Pitta.

Diuretics

Western: Used to increase the flow of urine; for water retention, edema and cystitis.
Comments: Some of these herbs are used for conditions of accumulated and congested Fluids such as edema. Other, more Cooling herbs are used for Damp-Heat conditions such as cystitis.
Western Herbal Examples:
Cooling:

- Cleavers, aerial parts, *Galium aparine*
- Coriander, leaf, seed, *Coriandrum sativum*
- Cornsilk, stylus, *Zea mays*
- Dandelion, leaf, *Taraxacum officinale*
- Dianthus, aerial parts, *Dianthus chinensis*
- Horsetail, aerial parts, *Equisetum spp.*
- Lysimachia, aerial parts, *Lysimachia christinae*
- Nettles, leaf, *Urtica dioica*
- Pipsissewa, aerial parts, *Chimaphila umbellata*
- Plantago, seed, *Plantago asiatica*
- Plantain, root, *Alisma plantago*
- Poria, sclerotium, *Poria cocos*
- Uva Ursi, leaves, *Arctostaphylos uva ursi*
- Watermelon, seed, *Citrullus lanatus*

Warming:

- Buchu, leaf, *Agathosma betulia*
- Parsley, seeds, leaf, root, *Petroselinum crispum*
- Watercress, flower, leaf, *Nasturtium officinalis*

Chemical Constituents: Varies
Phases: Earth, Water, Air, Space
Taste: Sweet, Bitter
Functional Principle: Cool
Chinese Medicine: Herbs that Drain Dampness
Ayurveda: Herbs that reduce Kapha and Pitta

Emetics

Western: Used to induce vomiting.
Comments: The main function of these herbs is to expel mucus and Phlegm by vomiting. This treatment is used therapeutically in Ayurveda for hardy Kapha constitutions only.
Western Herbal Examples:

- Black Cohosh, root, *Cimicifuga racemosa*
- Lobelia, seed, flower, leaf, *Lobelia inflata*

Chemical Constituents: Bitter compounds
Phases: Space, Air
Taste: Bitter
Functional Principle: Cold
Chinese Medicine: Herbs That Expel Phlegm by Inducing Vomiting
Ayurveda: Herbs that decrease Kapha

Emmenagogues

Western: Used to promote menstruation. These herbs may also be used as tonics for the female reproductive system.
Comments: To promote menstruation; some herbs are used to move stagnation due to Blood/Qi deficiency. As tonics some herbs are used to nourish due to Yin deficiency.
Western Herbal Examples:

- Blue Cohosh, root, *Caulophyllum thalictroides*
- Curcuma, rhizome, tuber, *Curcuma longa*
- Calendula, flower, *Calendula officinalis*
- Frankincense, resin, *Boswellia carterii*
- Lovage, root, *Ligusticum levisticum*
- Motherwort, aerial parts, *Leonurus heterophyllus*
- Myrrh, resin, *Commiphora myrrha*
- Peach Kernel, seed, *Prunus persica, spp.*
- Peony (Red), root, *Paeoniae rubra*
- Pennyroyal, aerial parts, *Mentha pulegium*
- Rose, flower, *Rosa rugosa*
- Rue, aerial parts, *Ruta graveolens*
- Safflower, flower, *Carthamus tinctorius*
- Sage, root, *Salvia miltiorrhiza*
- Tansy, flower, *Tanacetum vulgare*
- Vervain, aerial parts, *Verbena officinalis*

Chemical Constituents: Polysaccharides
Phases: Water, Earth
Taste: Sweet
Functional Principle: Cool
Chinese Medicine: Herbs that Tonify the Blood; Herbs that Tonify the Yin
Ayurveda: Herbs that increase Kapha

Notes

Notes

Emollients

Western: Applied externally, these soften and soothe the skin.
Comments: These herbs are similar to Demulcents.
Western Herbal Examples:

- Chickweed, aerial parts, *Stellaria media*
- Comfrey, leaf, root, *Symphytum officinale*
- Flax, seed, *Linum usitatissimum*
- Oats, seed, *Avena sativa*
- Slippery Elm, inner bark, *Ulmus fulva*

Chemical Constituents: Polysaccharides
Phases: Water, Earth
Taste: Sweet
Functional Principle: Cool
Chinese Medicine: Herbs that Tonify Yin
Ayurveda: Herbs that increase Kapha; reduce Vata and Pitta

Expectorants

Western: Used to help expel excess mucus from the lungs.
Comments: These herbs dry and/or thin excess mucus/Phlegm in the Lung-System. By eliminating and thinning the excess mucus/Phlegm, the coughing will abate by allowing the Lung-Qi to move downward in its normal pattern.
Western Herbal Examples:

- Apricot, seed, *Prunus armeniaca*
- Aster, root, *Aster tataricus*
- Coltsfoot, flower, *Tussilago farfara*
- Lungwort, root, *Pulminaria officinalis*
- Mulberry, bark, *Morus alba*
- Mullein, flower, leaf, root, *Verbascum thapsus*
- Wild Cherry, bark, *Prunus avium*

Chemical Constituents: Varies
Phases: Air, Fire
Taste: Pungent
Functional Principle: Warm
Chinese Medicine: Herbs that Relieve Coughing and Wheezing
Ayurveda: Herbs that reduce Kapha

Febrifuges

Western: Used to reduce fever.
Comments: These herbs are similar to Antipyretics.
Western Herbal Examples: See Antipyretics.
Chemical Constituents: Varies
Phases: Space, Air, Water, Earth
Taste: Bitter, Sweet

Functional Principle: Cold
Chinese Medicine: Herbs that Drain Fire
Ayurveda: Herbs that reduce Pitta

Galactagogues

Western: Used to increase the production of breast milk.
Comments: These herbs nourish Fluids.
Western Herbal Examples:

- Anise, seed, *Pimpinella anisum*
- Blessed Thistle, aerial parts, *Cnicus benedictus*
- Fennel, fruit, *Foeniculum vulgare*
- Fenugreek, seed, *Trigonella foenum-graecum*
- Raspberry, fruit, *Rubus chingii*

Chemical Constituents: Polysaccharides
Phases: Water, Earth
Taste: Sweet
Functional Principle: Cool
Chinese Medicine: Herbs That Tonify Yin
Ayurveda: Herbs that increase Kapha; reduce Vata

Hemostatics

Western: Used to stop hemorrhaging and internal bleeding.
Comments: See Astringents.
Western Herbal Examples:

- Agrimony, aerial parts, *Agrimonia pilosa*
- Burnet, root, *Sanguisorba officinalis*
- Cattail, pollen, *Typha angustifolia*
- Madder, root, *Rubia cordifolia*
- Mugwort, leaf, *Artemisia argyi*
- Raspberry, leaf, *Rubus chingii*
- Shepherd's Purse, aerial parts, *Capsella bursa-pastoris*

Chemical Constituents: Tannins
Phases: Air, Earth
Taste: Astringent
Functional Principle: Cool
Chinese Medicine: Herbs that Stabilize and Bind
Ayurveda: Herbs that calm Pitta and Kapha

Hepatics

Western: Used to aid the liver by toning and strengthening; increases the flow of bile.
Comments: See Bitters.

Notes

Notes

Western Herbal Examples:

- Dandelion, root, *Taraxacum officinale*
- Goldenseal, root, *Hydrastis canadensis*
- Oregon Grape, root, *Mahonia repens*
- Wild Yam, root, *Dioscorea villosa*
- Yellowdock, root, *Rumex crispus*

Chemical Constituents: Varies
Phases: Acrid, Bitter
Taste: Air, Earth, Water, Fire
Functional Principle: Varies
Chinese Medicine: Herbs that Regulate Qi
Ayurveda: Herbs that reduce Pitta

Laxatives

Western: Used to promote bowel movements.
Comments: Laxatives are less drastic than purgatives and are moistening. See also Cathartics and Purgatives.
Western Herbal Examples:

- Cannabis, seed, *Cannabis sativa*
- Castor, seed oil, *Ricinus communis*
- Plum, fruit, *Prunus japonica*

Chemical Constituents: Varies
Phases: Water, Earth, Air, Space
Taste: Sweet, Bitter
Functional Principle: Cool
Chinese Medicine: Herbs that Drain Downward
Ayurveda: Herbs that increase Vata

Lithotropics

Western: Used to prevent and eliminate urinary, gallbladder, and kidney stones and gravel.
Comments: In Eastern medicine urinary and gallbladder stones are considered Phlegm accumulation due to stagnation. See Anticatarrhals.
Western Herbal Examples:
For urinary stones:

- Buchu, leaf, *Agathosma betulia*
- Cleavers, aerial parts, *Galium aparine*
- Cornsilk, stylus, *Zea mays*
- Dandelion, root, *Taraxacum officinale*
- Gravel Root, root, *Eupatorium purpureum*
- Marshmallow, root, *Althea officinalis*
- Parsley, root, *Petroselinum crispum*
- Gravel Root, root, *Eupatorium purpureum*

Notes

For gallbladder stones:

- Cascara, bark, *Cascara sagrada*
- Oregon Grape, root, *Mahonia repens*

For kidney stones:

- Dandelion, root, *Taraxacum officinale*
- Gravel Root, root, *Eupatorium purpureum*
- Nettles, leaf, *Urtica dioica*
- Parsley, root, *Petroselinum crispum*

Chemical Constituents: Varies
Phases: Air, Space, Water, Earth, Fire
Taste: Bitter, Sweet, Acrid
Functional Principle: Varies
Chinese Medicine: Cool/Warm Herbs that Transform Phlegm-Cold/Heat
Ayurveda: Herbs that reduce Kapha, Pitta

Nervines

Western: Used to calm, strengthen and tone the nervous system.
Comments: These herbs help with nervous conditions such as irritability, anxiety, and insomnia and have either a nourishing and cooling effect or a warming effect. The minerals have a heavy downward effect to calm the nervous system, but they do not affect the level of consciousness.
Western Herbal Examples:

Minerals:

- Amber, stone, *Succinum*
- Dragon Bone, bone, *Draconis*
- Hematite, mineral
- Magnetite, mineral
- Oyster, shell, *Ostrea gigas*
- Pearl, *Pteria margaritifera*

Cooling:

- Arbor-Vitae, leafy twig, *Biota orientalis*
- California Poppy, aerial parts, *Eschscholzia californica*
- Chamomile, flower, *Matricaria chamomilla; Anthemis nobilis*
- Hops, strobili, *Humulus lupulus*
- Lady's Slipper, root, *Cypripedium acaule*
- Passion Flower, flower, *Passiflora incarnata*
- Scullcap, aerial parts, *Scutellaria laterifolia*
- Wood Betony, aerial parts, *Betonica officinalis*

Warming:

- Kava, root, *Piper methysticum*
- Valerian, root, *Valeriana officinalis*

Chemical Constituents: polysaccharides
Phases: Earth, Water
Taste: Sweet

Notes

Functional Principle: Varies
Chinese Medicine: Herbs that Nourish the Heart and Calm the Spirit, Substances that Anchor Settle, and Calm the Spirit
Ayurveda: Herbs that reduce Vata

Parasiticides see Anthelmintics

Pectorals

Western: Used to promote a healing and strengthening effect on the respiratory system.
Comments: These herbs nourish and/or moisten the Lungs, that is they Tonify the Lung-Yin.
Western Herbal Examples:

- Coltsfoot, leaf, flower, *Tussilago farfara*
- Comfrey, leaf, root, *Symphytum officinale*
- Elecampane, root, *Inula japonica*
- Mullein, flower, leaf, root, *Verbascum thapsus*
- Licorice, root, *Glycyrrhiza glabra*

Chemical Constituents: Polysaccharides
Phases: Water, Earth
Taste: Sweet
Functional Principle: Cool
Chinese Medicine: Herbs that Tonify Yin
Ayurveda: Herbs that increase Kapha; reduce Pitta

Purgatives

Western: These are used for constipation with accumulation of Heat.
Comments: These herbs are cold in nature to clear accumulated Heat. See also: Cathartics and Laxatives.
Western Herbal Examples:

- Aloe, leaf, *Aloe vera*
- Buckthorn, bark, *Rhamnus cathartica*
- Cascara, bark, *Cascara sagrada*
- Epsom Salts, *Mirabilitum*
- Rhubarb, root, *Rheum palmatum*
- Senna, leaf, *Cassia angustifolia*

Chemical Constituents: Varies
Phases: Space, Air
Taste: Bitter
Functional Principle: Cold
Chinese Medicine: Downward Draining Herbs: Purgatives
Ayurveda: Herbs that reduce Pitta

Rubefacients

Notes

Western: When applied to the skin, these herbs stimulate the dilation of the capillaries and can cause local irritation thereby drawing inflammation and congestion from deeper tissues. Also used to increase circulation and promote surface warming. They should be used with moistening herbs that minimize skin irritation.

Western Herbal Examples:

- Capsicum, fruit, *Capsicum frutescens*
- Clove, flower bud, *Caryopyhllus aromaticus*
- Ginger, rhizome, *Zingiberis officinalis*
- Horseradish, root, *Amoracia rusticana*
- Mustard, seed, *Brassica alba*

Chemical Constituents: Volatile oils
Phases: Air, Fire
Taste: Pungent
Functional Principle: Warm
Chinese Medicine: Substances for External Application
Ayurveda: Herbs that reduce Vata, Kapha, increase Pitta

Sedatives

Western: Used to help cope with stress and nervous disorders; also as an aid for sleep; promotes calmness.
Comments: See Nervines, Aromatics Herbs that Open the Orifices.
Chemical Constituents: Polysaccharides
Phases: Earth, Water
Taste: Sweet
Functional Principle: Varies
Chinese Medicine: Herbs that Calm the Spirit
Ayurveda: Herbs that reduce Vata

Sialagogues

Western: Used to stimulate the secretion of saliva to aid digestion.
Comments: See Bitters and Hepatics.
Western Herbal Examples:

- Capsicum, fruit, *Capsicum frutescens*
- Echinacea, root, *Echinacea spp.*
- Gentian, root, *Gentiana lutea*
- Ginger, rhizome, *Zingiberis officinalis*
- Pepper, fruit, *Piper nigrum*

Chemical Constituents: Varies
Phases: Air, Space, Fire
Taste: Bitter, Pungent
Functional Principle: Varies

Notes

Chinese Medicine: Herbs that Regulate Qi
Ayurveda: Herbs that increase Pitta

Soporifics

Western: Used to induce sleep.
Comments: See Nervines and Sedatives.
Western Herbal Examples: See Nervines and Sedatives.
Chemical Constituents: Polysaccharides
Phases: Earth, Water
Taste: Sweet
Functional Principle: Varies
Chinese Medicine: Herbs that Calm the Spirit
Ayurveda: Herbs that reduce Vata

Stimulants

Western: Used to increase Qi-energy in the body by increasing metabolism.
Comments: Depending on the symptoms, the condition of poor metabolism could be a faulty functioning or stagnant digestive system or systemic weakness due to various factors, therefore, different herbs would be used depending on the condition being treated. See also Bitters, Hepatics, and Sialagogues.
Western Herbal Examples:

- Bayberry, bark, *Myrica cerifera*
- Capsicum, fruit, *Capsicum frutescens*
- Cinnamon, bark, *Cinnamon cassia*
- Clove, flower bud, *Caryophyllus aromaticus*
- Fennel, fruit, *Foeniculum vulgare*
- Ginger, rhizome, *Zingiberis officinalis*
- Horseradish, root, *Amoracia rusticana*
- Mustard, seed, *Brassica alba*
- Pepper, fruit, *Piper nigrum*
- Prickly Ash, bark, *Zanthoxylum americanum*

Chemical Constituents: Varies
Phases: Air, Fire, Water, Earth
Taste: Pungent, Sweet
Functional Principle: Warm
Chinese Medicine: Herbs that Warm the Interior and Expel Cold
Ayurveda: Herbs that reduce Vata and Kapha

Styptics

Western: Used to reduce or stop external bleeding by their astringent and/or coagulating effects.

Comments: There are many patterns of external bleeding of which trauma is only one. For example, nosebleeds could be caused by Heat. See Hemostatics.

Western Herbal Examples:

- Cattail, pollen, *Typha angustifolia*
- Shepherd's Purse, aerial parts, *Capsella bursa-pastoris*
- Spider Webs
- Yarrow, flower, leaf, *Achillea millefolium*

Chemical Constituents: Varies
Phases: Air, Earth
Taste: Acrid, Astringent
Functional Principle: Varies
Chinese Medicine: Herbs that Stop Bleeding/Substances for External Application
Ayurveda: Herbs that reduce Kapha

Notes

Sudorifics

Western: Used to produce profuse perspiration when taken hot.
Comments: These herbs are used to dislodge a pathogenic factor that has not yet penetrated the body such as Wind-Heat, Wind-Cold, and Wind-Damp. These are the first symptoms of a cold or flu such as chills, fever, headache, muscle aches, and some rashes. Opening the pores to promote sweating expels the pathogen. See Diaphoretics.

Western Herbal Examples:

- Elder, flower, *Sambucus nigra*
- Hyssop, aerial parts, *Hyssopus officinalis*
- Peppermint, aerial parts, *Mentha piperita*

Chemical Constituents: varies
Phases: Air, Earth, Fire
Taste: Acrid
Functional Principle: Warm
Chinese Medicine: Warm Herbs that Release the Exterior
Ayurveda: Herbs that reduce Kapha

Tonics

Western: Used to strengthen (Yang aspect) and nourish (Yin aspect) specific organs of the body. Most tonics have general effects on the whole body and, specific effects on various organs.
Comments: In Eastern medicine these herbs are further delineated into the origin of the condition, that is, whether the condition is one of Yin, Yang, Qi, or Blood deficiency. For example, if the condition is one of exhaustion it could be due to Yang deficiency (similar to adrenal insufficiency) or Yin deficiency of which there is no parallel in Western derived thought including Western herbal medicine. Unfortunately, the lack of differentiation in the Western view usually leads to strengthening the Yang when often the Yin should be nourished. This lack of awareness can lead to the condition not improving to making the condition worse. See also Demulcents, Vulneraries.

Notes

Western Herbal Examples:

Tonify Qi:

- American Ginseng, root, *Panax quinquefolium*
- Astragalus, root, *Astragalus membranaceus*
- Elecampane, root, *Inula japonica*
- Ginseng, root, *Panax ginseng*
- Licorice, root, *Glycyrrhiza glabra*
- Spikenard, root, *Aralia racemosa*
- Siberian Ginseng, root, *Eleutherococcus senticosus*
- Solomon Seal, rhizome, *Polygonatum sibiricum*

Tonify Yang:

- Ashwagandha, root, *Withania somnifera*
- Astragalus, seed, *Astragalus complanatus*
- Cardamom, Black, fruit, *Alpinia oxyphylla*
- Damiana, leaf, *Turner aphrodisiaca*
- Dodder, seed, *Cuscuta chinensis*
- Epimedium, aerial parts, *Epimedium grandiflorum*
- False Unicorn, root, *Chamaelirium luteum*
- Fenugreek, seed, *Trigonella foenum-graecum*
- Leek, seed, *Allium tuberosum*
- Saw Palmetto, fruit, *Sabal serrulata*
- Walnut, seed, *Juglans regia*

Tonify Yin:

- American Ginseng, root, *Panax quinquefolium*
- Asparagus, tuber, *Asparagus cochinchinensis*
- Lily, bulb, *Lilium brownii*
- Marshmallow, root, *Althea officinalis*
- Sesame, seed, *Sesamum indicum*
- Slippery Elm, inner bark, *Ulmus fulva*
- Solomon Seal, rhizome, *Polygonatum sibiricum*

Chemical Constituents: Polysaccharides
Phases: Water, Earth, Fire
Taste: Sweet, Salty
Functional Principle: Varies
Chinese Medicine: Herbs That Tonify the Qi, Herbs that Tonify the Yin, Herbs That Tonify Yang
Ayurveda: Herbs that increase Kapha or Pitta

Vulneraries

Western: Used to help heal the body by promoting cellular growth and repair.
Comments: These herbs are nourishing and moistening and are used to treat a lack of Essential Fluids in the organ-systems resulting in Yin deficiency a condition where the lack of Essential Fluids results in the appearance of too much Heat. See Demulcents, Tonics.

Western Herbal Examples:

- Aloe, leaf, *Aloe vera*
- Comfrey, leaf, root, *Symphytum officinale*
- Chickweed, aerial parts, *Stellaria media*
- Calendula, flower, *Calendula officinalis*
- Plantain, root, *Alisma plantago*
- St. John's Wort, aerial parts, *Hypericum perforatum*

Chemical Constituents: Polysaccharides

Phases: Water, Earth

Taste: Sweet

Functional Principle: Cool

Chinese Medicine: Herbs That Tonify Yin

Ayurveda: Herbs that increase Kapha, reduce Pitta, Vata.

Notes

Table–13-2

THE TASTES & THEIR PHASES

The larger X is the predominant Phase

TASTE	SPACE	AIR	FIRE	WATER	EARTH
SWEET				x	X
SOUR			X		x
SALTY			X	x	
PUNGENT		x	X		
BITTER	x	X			
ASTRINGENT		X			x
ACRID	X	x	x		
BLAND		x			X

Notes

Table–13-3

WESTERN THERAPEUTICS & THEIR PREDOMINANT PHASES

The larger X is the predominant Phase

WESTERN ACTION	SPACE	AIR	FIRE	WATER	EARTH
Alterative	x	**X**			
Analgesic		**X**	**X**	**X**	**X**
Antacid	x	**X**		**X**	**X**
Anthelmintic	x	**X**	**X**		
Anti-asthmatic		**X**	**X**	**X**	**X**
Antibiotic	**X**	x			
Anti-pyretic	**X**	x			
Anti-septic	**X**	x	x		
Anti-spasmodic			x	**X**	**X**
Astringent		**X**			x
Bitter	x	**X**			
Carminative		x	**X**		
Cathartic	**X**	x		**X**	**X**
Cholagogues	**X**	x		**X**	
Demulcents				**X**	x
Diaphoretics	x	**X**	**X**		
Diuretics	x	**X**			**X**
Emetics	x	**X**			
Emmenagogues		x	x	**X**	**X**

Notes

WESTERN ACTION	SPACE	AIR	FIRE	WATER	EARTH
Emollients				X	x
Expectorants		X	x		
Febrifuges	X	x			
Galactagogues		X		x	X
Hepatics	x	X			
Hemostatics		X			x
Laxatives	x	X		x	X
Lithotropics	x	X		x	X
Nervines			x	x	X
Pectorals				X	x
Rubefacients		x	X		
Sedatives				x	X
Sialagogues		x	X	X	
Stimulants		X	x		
Soporifics				x	X
Styptics		x			X
Sudorifics		X	x		X
Tonics			x	X	x
Vulneraries				X	x

Notes

Chapter 14:

Quanta of the Trade: *Materia Medica*

This chapter is not intended as a comprehensive *Materia Medica* but as a listing of Western and some Eastern herbs that are often used in the different categories of Western herbal Medicine along with their Functional Principles and organ-systems, for which the herb has an affinity in addition to the part of the plant used. This information is for the Western herbal practitioner or medical doctor who would like to have more consistent results provided by thousands of years of expertise of Eastern Medicine. Included in the information for each herb, is the category of an herb's ability to target specific organ-systems. This gives the practitioner more information as to how to use the herb more effectively.

The Eastern herbs will have their *pin yin* name listed although there are many herbs used by both Eastern and Western traditions.

Table–14-1

TASTES & CORRESPONDING ORGANS

TASTE	ORGAN
Sour	Liver
Acrid	Lungs
Bitter	Heart
Salty	Kidneys
Sweet	Metabolic

For ease of reference for the Western student, the botanical names (genus and species) for the herbs are cited as opposed to the pharmaceutical name which is commonly used in Eastern medicine.

For additional information about the herbs, please consult the *Chinese Herbal Medicine Materia Medica* by Bensky and Gamble and/or *Planetary Herbology* by Michael Tierra.

Notes

Table–14-2

WESTERN—EASTERN CATEGORY EQUIVALENTS

WESTERN CATEGORY	EASTERN CATEGORY and Subcategory
Alteratives	Clear Heat—Cool the Blood
Analgesics	Extinguish Wind and Stop Tremors
Anodynes	Extinguish Wind and Stop Tremors
Antacids	Clear Heat—Drain Fire
Anthelmintics	Expel Parasites
Antiasthmatics	Transform Phlegm and Stop Coughing—Relieve Coughing and Wheezing
Anticatarrhals	Transform Phlegm and Stop Coughing
Antibiotics	Clear Heat—Clear Heat and Resolve Toxicity
Antimicrobial	Clear Heat—Clear Heat and Resolve Toxicity
Antipyretics	Clear Heat
Antiseptics	Clear Heat—Clear Heat and Resolve Toxicity
Anti-rheumatics	Dispel Wind-Dampness
Anti-spasmodics	Extinguish Wind and Stop Tremors
Astringents	Stabilize and Bind
Bitters	Regulate the Qi
Carminatives	Aromatics that Transform Dampness
Cholagogues	Downward Draining
Demulcents	Tonify—Tonify Yin
Diaphoretics	Release the Exterior
Digestants	Regulate the Qi
Diuretics	Drain Dampness
Emetics	Expel Phlegm by Inducing Vomiting
Emmenagogues	Tonify—Tonify Yin/Blood
Emollients	Tonify—Tonify Yin
Expectorants	Transform Phlegm and Stop Coughing—Relieve Coughing and Wheezing
Febrifuges	Clear Heat—Drain Fire
Galactagogues	Tonify—Tonify Yin

Notes

WESTERN CATEGORY	EASTERN CATEGORY and Subcategory
Hemostatics	Stabilize and Bind
Hepatics	Regulate the Qi
Laxatives	Downward Draining
Lithotropics	Transform Phlegm
Nervines	Calm the Spirit
Parasiticides	Expel Parasites
Pectorals	Tonify—Tonify Yin
Rubefacients	External Application
Sedatives	Calm the Spirit
Sialagogues	Regulate the Qi
Soporifics	Calm the Spirit
Stimulants	Warm Interior and Expel Cold
Styptics	Regulate the Blood—Stop Bleeding
Sudorifics	Release the Exterior
Tonics	Tonify
Vulnerary	Tonify—Tonify Yin

Antipyretics—Herbs that Clear Heat

In Eastern Medicine, Heat refers to any condition that exhibits heat signs such as fevers, dryness of the throat, mouth, eyes, stool, red coloration on the skin or eyes, yellow tongue coat, or dark yellow and scanty urine. There are several Antipyretic categories: Herbs that Cool the Blood, Herbs that Clear Heat and Resolve Toxicity, Herbs that Drain Fire, Herbs that Clear Heat and Dry Dampness, and Herbs that Clear Heat from Deficiency.

If there is an exterior Heat pattern use Cooling Herbs That Release the Exterior.

Alteratives—Herbs that Cool the Blood

These herbs are used when there is Heat in the Blood with symptoms such as rashes, nosebleeds, vomiting or coughing of blood, and blood in the urine or stool. The excess Heat in the Blood creates a condition of increased permeability of the capillaries resulting in bleeding.[1]

The main Phases are Space and Air for cooling and Water and Earth for nourishing the Blood and Essential Fluids or Yin. The main Tastes are Bitter and Sweet.

These herbs reduce Pitta.

- **Burdock—Arctium lappa, root, *niu bang zi***
  Functional Principle: bitter, sweet, cool
  Organ-System: Lungs, Stomach, Kidneys, Liver

Notes

- **Dandelion Root—Taraxacum officinale, root**
  Functional Principle: bitter, sweet, cool
  Organ-System: Liver, Stomach

- **Honeysuckle—Lonicera japonica, flower, *jin yin hua***
  Functional Principle: sweet, bitter, cold
  Organ-System: Lungs, Stomach

- **Red Clover—Trifolium pretense, flower**
  Functional Principle: sweet, salty, cool
  Organ-System: Liver, Heart, Lungs

- **Rehmannia—Rehmannia glutinosa, root, *sheng di huang***
  Functional Principle: sweet, bitter, cold
  Organ-System: Heart, Kidneys, Liver

Antibiotics, Antimicrobial, Antiseptics or Herbs that Clear Heat and Resolve Toxicity

These herbs are used to help clear viral and bacterial infections such as flu, infected sores, and abscesses.

The main Phases are Space and Air for their cooling and dispersing actions.

These herbs reduce Pitta.

- **Andrographitis—Andrographis paniculata, herb, *chuan xin lian***
  Functional Principle: bitter, cold
  Organ-System: Large Intestine Lungs, Small Intestine, Stomach

- **Begonia—Begonia spp., herb, *zi bei tian kui***
  Functional Principle: sweet, cool
  Organ-System: Liver, Stomach

- **Chaparral—Larrea tridentata, leaf**
  Functional Principle: acrid, bitter, salty, cool
  Organ-System: Kidneys, Lungs, Liver

- **Chrysanthemum Flowers—Chrysanthemum indicum, flower, *ju hua***
  Functional Principle: bitter, acrid, cold
  Organ-System: Lungs, Liver

- **Dandelion—Taraxacum officinale, leaf, root, *pu gong ying***
  Functional Principle: bitter, sweet, cold
  Organ-System: Liver, Stomach

Notes

- **Echinacea—Echinacea spp., root**
  Functional Principle: bitter, pungent, cool
  Organ-System: Lungs, Stomach, Liver

- **Forsythia—Forsythia suspensa, fruit, *lian qiao***
  Functional Principle: bitter, acrid, cold
  Organ-System: Heart, Liver, Gall Bladder

- **Goldenseal—Hydrastis canadensis, rhizome**
  Functional Principle: bitter, cold
  Organ-System: Heart, Liver, Stomach, Large Intestine

- **Honeysuckle—Lonicera japonica, flower, *jin yin hua***
  Functional Principle: sweet, bitter, cold
  Organ-System: Lungs, Stomach

- **Iris—Iris versicolor, rhizome**
  Functional Principle: acrid, bitter, cold
  Organ-System: Liver, Gall Bladder, Large Intestine, Stomach

- **Pulsatilla—Anemone pulsatilla, root, *bai tou weng***
  Functional Principle: bitter, cold
  Organ-System: Large Intestine, Liver, Stomach

- **Purslane—Portulacea oleracea, aerial part, *ma chi xian***
  Functional Principle: sour, cold
  Organ-System: Large Intestine, Liver

- **Usnea—Usnea spp., whole plant**
  Functional Principle: sweet, cold
  Organ-System: Lungs, Liver, Large Intestine

- **Violet—Viola odorata, tricolor, whole plant, *zi hua di ding***
  Functional Principle: sweet, bitter, cool
  Organ-System: Lungs, Stomach, Liver, Heart

Febrifuges or Herbs that Drain Fire

These are extremely Cold herbs and can be used to treat high fevers.

The main Phases are Space and Air for their cold properties and Water and Earth for their cooling and moistening qualities. The moistening qualities help cool the Blood so important in high fevers.

These herbs reduce Pitta.

Notes

- **Celosia—Celosia argentea, seed, *qing xiang zi***
  Functional Principle: sweet, cool
  Organ-System: Liver

- **Gardenia—Gardenia jasminoidis, flower, *zhi zi***
  Functional Principle: bitter, cold
  Organ-System: Heart, Liver, Stomach, Triple Burner

- **Gypsum—Calcium sulfate, *shi gao***
  Functional Principle: sweet, acrid, very cold
  Organ-System: Stomach, Lungs

- **Self Heal—Prunella vulgaris, flower bud, *xia ku cao***
  Functional Principle: bitter, acrid, cold
  Organ-System: Gall Bladder, Liver

- **Violet—Viola odorata, tricolor, whole plant, *zi hua di ding***
  Functional Principle: sweet, bitter, cool
  Organ-System: Lungs, Stomach, Liver, Heart

Herbs That Clear Heat and Dry Dampness

These herbs are used for conditions of Damp-Heat in the lower body, such as prostate, vaginal, or urinary infections, and diarrhea due to intestinal bacteria or amoebic infection, rashes or heat in the genital area.

The main Phases of these herbs are Space and Air.

- **Barberry root—Berberis vulgaris, root bark**
  Functional Principle: bitter, cold
  Organ-System: Liver, Stomach, Large Intestine

- **Bitterroot—Lewisia rediviva, root**
  Functional Principle: bitter, sweet, cool
  Organ-System: Liver, Metabolic

- **Cinchona—Cinchona officinalis, bark**
  Functional Principle: bitter, cold
  Organ-System: Stomach, Heart, Liver

- **Gentian—Gentiana lutea, root, *long dan cao***
  Functional Principle: bitter, cold
  Organ-System: Liver, Gall Bladder, Stomach

Notes

- **Goldenseal—Hydrastis canadensis, rhizome**
  Functional Principle: bitter, cold
  Organ-System: Heart, Liver, Stomach, Large Intestine

- **Oregon Grape—Mahonia repens, root bark**
  Functional Principle: bitter, cold
  Organ-System: Liver, Stomach, Large Intestine

- **Poplar—Populus spp., leaf, bark**
  Functional Principle: bitter, cold
  Organ-System: Large Intestine, Lungs, Stomach

- **Scutellaria—Scutellaria baicalensis, root, *huang qin***
  Functional Principle: bitter, cold
  Organ-System: Gall Bladder, Large Intestine, Lungs, Stomach

- **Wahoo—Euonymus atropurpureus, bark and root**
  Functional Principle: bitter, cold
  Organ-System: Lungs, Liver, Gall Bladder, Stomach

- **Willow Bark—Salix nigra, bark, flower**
  Functional Principle: bitter, cold
  Organ-System: Liver, Kidneys, Heart

Herbs That Clear Heat from Deficiency

These herbs are used when the Essential Fluids have been damaged due to intense or long-term Heat and sweating in the body known as Summerheat in Chinese Medicine. Some symptoms in this category would be afternoon or evening feverishness, heat in the palms and soles, and a red tongue with little coating.

The main Phases of these herbs are Earth and Water for their moistening qualities to counter the drying effects of heat.

- **Artemisia—Artemisia annua, aerial part, *qing hao***
  Functional Principle: bitter, cold
  Organ-System: Kidneys, Liver, Gall Bladder

- **Borage—Borago officinalis, leaf**
  Functional Principle: bitter, sweet, cool
  Organ-System: Lungs, Heart

- **Hibiscus—Hibiscus rosa sinensis, flower**
  Functional Principle: sour, sweet, cool
  Organ-System: Liver, Stomach

Notes

- **Lycii—Lycii, bark, *di gu pi***
  Functional Principle: sweet, bland, cold
  Organ-System: Lungs, Liver, Kidneys

- **Stellaria—Stellaria dichotoma, root, *yin chai hu***
  Functional Principle: sweet, cool
  Organ-System: Liver, Stomach

Diaphoretics or Herbs That Release the Exterior

These herbs are used to dislodge a pathogenic factor that has not yet penetrated into the interior of the body such as Wind-Heat, Wind-Cold, or Wind-Damp, which are the first symptoms of a cold or flu such as chills, fever, headache, muscle aches, and some rashes. They help open the pores to induce sweating, which usually expels the pathogen. Additional help may be needed by using this category of herbs especially if the pathogen has moved into the deeper layer of the muscles. The Functional Principle of this category of herbs varies depending on whether the Functional Principle of the condition is one of Heat or Cold. Using the wrong herbs at the wrong time can make the condition worse.

Warming Diaphoretics or Herbs That Release the Exterior

These herbs dispel exterior Wind-Cold and are used when there are predominant chills and a slight fever. There could be symptoms of headache, body aches and stiffness, and stiff neck or neck pain.

The main Phases of this category of herbs are Air and Fire. The main Taste is Pungent. The Fire Phase along with the Air Phase disperses the exterior Cold.

These herbs calm Vata and Kapha doshas with their warming qualities and will, therefore, increase Pitta dosha.

- **Angelica dahurica, root, *bai zhi***
  Functional Principle: acrid, bitter, warm
  Organ-System: Lungs, Stomach

- **Basil—Ocimum basilicum, leaf**
  Functional Principle: acrid, warm
  Organ-System: Lungs, Stomach

- **Cinnamon Twig—Cinnamon cassia, twig, *gui zhi***
  Functional Principle: pungent, sweet, warm
  Organ-System: Bladder, Lungs, Heart

- **Costmary—Tanacetum balsamita, leaf**
  Functional Principle: acrid, warm
  Organ-System: Stomach, Lungs

Notes

- **Ephedra—Ephedra sinica, aerial part, *ma huang***
  Functional Principle: acrid, bitter, warm
  Organ-System: Lungs, Bladder

- **Ginger Root—Zingiber officinale, root, *sheng jiang***
  Functional Principle: acrid, warm
  Organ-System: Lungs, Metabolic, Stomach

- **Hedge Nettle—Stachys palustris, leaf**
  Functional Principle: acrid, warm
  Organ-System: Lungs, Stomach

- **Hyssop—Hyssopus officinalis, whole plant**
  Functional Principle: acrid, warm
  Organ-System: Lungs, Stomach, Large Intestine, Bladder

- **Lovage—Ligusticum sinense, root, *gao ben***
  Functional Principle: acrid, warm
  Organ-System: Bladder

- **Magnolia Flowers—Magnolia officinalis, flower, *xin yi hua***
  Functional Principle: acrid, warm
  Organ-System: Lungs, Stomach

- **Marjoram—Origanum majorana, leaf**
  Functional Principle: acrid, warm
  Organ-System: Lungs, Stomach

- **Oregano—Organum vulgare, leaf**
  Functional Principle: acrid, warm
  Organ-System: Lungs, Stomach

- **Osha—Ligusticum porteri, root**
  Functional Principle: acrid, bitter, warm
  Organ-System: Lungs, Stomach

- **Sage—Salvia officinalis, leaf**
  Functional Principle: acrid, astringent, warm
  Organ-System: Lungs, Stomach

- **Savory—Satureja hortensis, whole plant**
  Functional Principle: acrid, bitter, warm
  Organ-System: Lungs, Stomach, Liver

Notes

- **Scallions—Allium pistulosum, bulb, *cong bai***
  Functional Principle: acrid, warm
  Organ-System: Lungs, Stomach

- **Wild Ginger—Asarum sieboldii, whole plant, *xi xin***
  Functional Principle: acrid, warm
  Organ-System: Lungs, Kidneys

- **Yerba Buena—Satureja douglasii, aerial part**
  Functional Principle: acrid, warm
  Organ-System: Lungs, Stomach, Bladder

Cooling Diaphoretics or Herbs That Release the Exterior

These herbs are used to treat exterior Wind-Heat with symptoms of fever and sore throat. There may also be slight chills.

The main Phases of this category are Air and Space that disperse and cool.

These herbs calm Pitta but can aggravate Vata and Kapha.

- **Black Cohosh—Cimicifuga spp., rhizome, *sheng ma***
  Functional Principle: sweet, acrid, cool
  Organ-System: Large Intestine, Lungs, Metabolic, Stomach

- **Bupleurum—Bupleurum chinense, root, *chai hu***
  Functional Principle: bitter, acrid, cool
  Organ-System: Gall Bladder, Liver, Pericardium, Triple Burner

- **Burdock Fruit—Arctium lappa, fruit, *niu bang zi***
  Functional Principle: acrid, bitter, cold
  Organ-System: Lungs, Stomach

- **Catnip—Nepeta cataria, leaf**
  Functional Principle: acrid, bitter
  Organ-System: Lungs, Liver

- **Chrysanthemum Flowers—Chrysanthemum indicum, flower, *ju hua***
  Functional Principle: bitter, acrid, cold
  Organ-System: Lungs, Liver

- **Elder Flowers—Sambucus nigra, flower**
  Functional Principle: acrid, bitter
  Organ-System: Lungs, Liver

Notes

- **Feverfew—Chrysanthemum parthenium, flower**
  Functional Principle: bitter, cool
  Organ-System: Stomach, Liver

- **Horsemint—Monarda haplocalycis, aerial part, *bo he***
  Functional Principle: acrid, aromatic, cool
  Organ-System: Lungs, Liver

- **Horsetail—Equisetum spp., aerial part, *mu zei***
  Functional Principle: sweet, bitter, neutral
  Organ-System: Liver, Lungs

- **Kudzu root—Pueraria lobata, root, *ge gen***
  Functional Principle: sweet, acrid, cool
  Organ-System: Metabolic, Stomach

- **Lemon Balm—Melissa officinalis, aerial part**
  Functional Principle: sour, acrid
  Organ-System: Lungs, Liver

- **Mulberry leaves—Morus alba, leaf, *sang ye***
  Functional Principle: sweet, bitter, cold
  Organ-System: Liver, Lungs

- **Peppermint—Mentha piperita, leaf**
  Functional Principle: acrid, bitter
  Organ-System: Lungs, Liver

- **Pleurisy root—Asclepias tuberosa, root**
  Functional Principle: bitter, acrid
  Organ-System: Lungs, Large Intestine, Heart

- **Vervain, blue—Verbena spp., aerial part**
  Functional Principle: bitter, cool
  Organ-System: Large Intestine, Lungs

- **Vitex Berries—Vitex spp., fruit, *man jing zi***
  Functional Principle: bitter, acrid, cool
  Organ-System: Bladder, Liver, Stomach

- **Yarrow—Achillea millefolium, aerial part**
  Functional Principle: bitter, acrid
  Organ-System: Lungs, Liver

Laxatives or Downward Draining Herbs

Downward draining herbs are those that either stimulate or lubricate the intestines to promote bowel movements. In Chinese Medicine there are three separate categories because of their very different actions: Purgatives, Demulcent Laxatives, and Cathartics.

These herbs increase Vata.

Notes

Purgatives

Purgatives are used when constipation is due to excess interior Heat or Heat-toxin.

The main Phases in this category are Space and Air which have cooling and moving qualities.

- **Aloe—Aloe spp., leaves, *lu hui***
  Functional Principle: bitter, cold
  Organ-System: Large Intestine, Liver, Stomach

- **Buckthorn Bark—Rhamnus catharticus, branch bark**
  Functional Principle: bitter, cold
  Organ-System: Stomach, Liver, Gall Bladder, Large Intestine

- **Butternut—Juglans cinerea, nigra, bark, root bark**
  Functional Principle: bitter, cold
  Organ-System: Large Intestine

- **Cascara Sagrada, branch bark**
  Functional Principle: bitter, cold
  Organ-System: Stomach, Liver, Gall Bladder, Small Intestine

- **Rhubarb root—Rheum palmatum, root and rhizome, *da huang***
  Functional Principle: bitter, cold
  Organ-System: Heart, Large Intestine, Liver, Stomach

- **Senna—Cassia spp., leaves, *fan xie ye***
  Functional Principle: sweet, bitter, cold
  Organ-System: Large Intestine

- **Walnut Bark—Juglans nigra, bark**
  Functional Principle: bitter, cold
  Organ-System: Large Intestine

Notes

Demulcent Laxatives

Laxatives are moistening herbs, usually seeds or nuts, to lubricate the intestines thereby promoting bowel movements.

The main Phases are Water and Earth that provide the moisture and Air and Space that provide the movement.

These herbs calm Vata.

- **Cannabis Seed—Cannabis sativa, seed, *huo ma ren***
  Functional Principle: sweet, neutral
  Organ-System: Large Intestine, Metabolic, Stomach

- **Flaxseed—Linum usitatissimum, seed**
  Functional Principle: sweet, neutral
  Organ-System: Metabolic, Large Intestine

- **Psyllium—Plantago psyllium, seed**
  Functional Principle: sweet, neutral
  Organ-System: Metabolic, Stomach, Large Intestine

Harsh Expellants—Cathartics

These herbs are used for constipation due to poor water metabolism where fluids have accumulated in the abdominal area. These are harsh and toxic substances and should only be used with caution.[2]

The main Phases for this category are Space and Air.

- **Elder Bark—Sambucus canadensis, bark**
  Functional Principle: bitter, toxic
  Organ-System: Stomach, Large Intestine

- **Mandrake Root—Mandragora spp., root**
  Functional Principle: bitter, cold, toxic
  Organ-System: Liver, Large Intestine

- **Morning Glory Seeds—Ipomoea spp., seed**
  Functional Principle: bitter, cold, toxic
  Organ-System: Lungs, Kidneys, Large Intestine, Small Intestine

- **Poke Root—Phytolacca acinosa, root, *shang lu***
  Functional Principle: bitter, cold
  Organ-System: Bladder, Kidneys, Large Intestine, Metabolic

- **Scotch Broom—Sarothamnus scoparius, tips**
  Functional Principle: bitter, cold, toxic
  Organ-System: Large Intestine, Kidneys

Notes

Diuretics or Herbs That Drain Dampness

There are several uses for these herbs. First are the herbs to reduce the accumulation of excess fluids in the lower body. Second are the herbs that deal with congested Fluids especially in the Lungs and Metabolic Systems. Third are the herbs that work with excess and stagnated Fluids combined with Heat symptoms such as fever, burning sensations, and yellow secretions.[3]

These herbs reduce Kapha and Pitta.

Cooling Herbs That Drain Dampness

- **Cleavers—Galium aparine, aerial part**
  Functional Principle: bitter, cool
  Organ-System: Bladder, Gall Bladder

- **Coriander—Coriandrum sativum, leaves**
  Functional Principle: acrid, neural, cool
  Organ-System: Bladder, Stomach

- **Cornsilk—Zea mays, stylus, *yu mi xu***
  Functional Principle: sweet, neutral
  Organ-System: Bladder, Gall Bladder, Liver

- **Dandelion Leaf—Taraxacum officinale, leaf**
  Functional Principle: bitter, cold
  Organ-System: Bladder, Liver

- **Dianthus—Dianthus chinensis, aerial part, *qu mai***
  Functional Principle: bitter, cold
  Organ-System: Bladder, Heart, Small Intestine

- **Gravel Root—Eupatorium purpureum, root**
  Functional Principle: bitter, acrid, neutral
  Organ-System: Kidneys, Gall Bladder, Bladder, Stomach, Liver

- **Horsetail—Equisetum spp., aerial part, *mu zei***
  Functional Principle: sweet, bitter, neutral
  Organ-System: Lungs, Liver

Notes

- **Hydrangea—Hydrangea arborescens, root**
  Functional Principle: acrid, cool
  Organ-System: Kidneys, Bladder, Large Intestine

- **Lysimachia—Lysimachia christina, aerial part, *jin qian cao***
  Functional Principle: sweet, bland, neutral
  Organ-System: Bladder, Gall Bladder, Kidneys, Liver

- **Nettles—Urtica dioica, aerial part**
  Functional Principle: bland, bitter, cool
  Organ-System: Small Intestine, Bladder, Lungs

- **Pellitory of the Wall—Parietaria judaica, aerial part**
  Functional Principle: acrid, cool
  Organ-System: Bladder, Kidneys, Large Intestine

- **Pipsissewa—Chimaphila umbellate, aerial part**
  Functional Principle: bitter, astringent, cool
  Organ-System: Heart, Bladder, Small Intestine, Metabolic

- **Plantain—Plantago spp., seed, *che qian zi***
  Functional Principle: sweet, cold
  Organ-System: Bladder, Kidneys, Liver, Lungs

- **Poria—Poria cocos, sclerotium, *fu ling***
  Functional Principle: sweet, bland, neutral
  Organ-System: Heart, Metabolic, Lungs

- **Uva Ursi—Arctostaphylos uva ursi, leaf**
  Functional Principle: bitter, astringent, cold
  Organ-System: Heart, Bladder, Small Intestine, Liver

- **Water Plantain—Alisma plantago, rhizome, *ze xie***
  Functional Principle: sweet, bland, cold
  Organ-System: Kidneys, Bladder

- **Watermelon Seeds—Citrullus lanatus, seed**
  Functional Principle: bland, neutral
  Organ-System: Bladder, Heart, Stomach

Warming Herbs That Drain Dampness

- **Buchu—Agathosma betulia, leaf**
  Functional Principle: pungent, warm
  Organ-System: Bladder, Stomach, Lungs

Notes

- **Parsley—Petroselinum crispum, leaf, root**
  Functional Principle: sweet, bland, warm
  Organ-System: Lungs, Stomach, Bladder, Liver

- **Watercress—Nasturtium officinalis, flower, leaf**
  Functional Principle: acrid, bitter, warm
  Organ-System: Kidneys, Bladder, Stomach, Lungs

Anti-Rheumatics or Herbs That Dispel Wind-Dampness

These herbs dispel Wind and Damp from the muscles, joints, and bones thereby alleviating pain and obstruction of Qi such as in arthritic conditions. There are four main types of painful obstruction:

- **Wind**—predominant where the pain moves from place to place
- **Cold**—predominant where there is reduced mobility of the joints and an aversion to cold
- **Damp**—predominant where there is fixed pain with swelling
- **Heat**—predominant where there is heat and swelling.[4]

There can be one or several of the above factors the Systems Herbalist needs to consider in order to clear each pathogenic factor involved.

Dispel Wind-Damp-Cold

These herbs have the main Phases of Space, Air for dispersing, Earth for drying and the Fire Phase for warming and penetrating. It should be noted that often Wind-Damp-Cold will present with some Heat from stagnation. In this case using cooling herbs will not provide relief or could make the condition worse as it will exacerbate the Cold condition. In that case this category of herbs is indicated.

These herbs calm Vata and Kapha.

Warming Herbs to Dispel Wind-Damp-Cold

- **Acanthopanacis—Acanthopanacis gracile, stylus, bark, *wu jia pi***
  Functional Principle: acrid, bitter, warm
  Organ-System: Kidneys, Liver

- **Birch—Betula spp., bark, leaf bud**
  Functional Principle: acrid, warm
  Organ-System: Stomach, Metabolic

Notes

- **Clematis—Clematis chinensis, root, *wei ling xian***
  Functional Principle: acrid, salty, warm
  Organ-System: Bladder

- **Cocklebur—Xanthium sibiricum, fruit, *cang er zi***
  Functional Principle: sweet, bitter, warm,
  Organ-System: Lungs

- **Kava—Piper methysticum, root**
  Functional Principle: pungent, bitter, warm
  Organ-System: Liver, Kidneys

- **Pine Wood—Pinus tabulaeformis, wood, *song jie***
  Functional Principle: bitter, warm
  Organ-System: Liver

- **Wintergreen—Gaultheria procumbens, leaf**
  Functional Principle: acrid, warm
  Organ-System: Liver, Lungs

Dispel Wind-Damp-Heat

These herbs have the Main Phases of Space and Air for dispersing and cooling, Earth for the drying quality and Fire for its penetrating quality. The Air and Fire Phases combined, or the Pungent Taste, is especially effective at penetrating the painful obstruction that cause the condition.

These herbs calm Pitta.

Cooling Herbs to Dispel Wind-Damp-Heat

- **Black Cohosh—Cimicifuga spp., rhizome, *sheng ma***
  Functional Principle: sweet, pungent, bitter, cool
  Organ-System: Liver, Metabolic, Stomach, Large Intestine

- **Devil's Claw—Harpagophytum procumbens, root**
  Functional Principle: bitter, cool
  Organ-System: Liver, Stomach

- **Meadowsweet—Filipendula ulmaria, aerial part**
  Functional Principle: bitter, astringent, cool
  Organ-System: Liver, Bladder, Large Intestine

- **Mulberry Twig—Morus alba, twig, *sang zhi***
  Functional Principle: bitter, sweet, cold
  Organ-System: Liver

Notes

- **Star Jasmine—Trachelospermum jasminoides, stem, *luo shi teng***
  Functional Principle: bitter, cold
  Organ-System: Liver

- **Yucca—Yucca spp., root**
  Functional Principle: sweet, bland, cool
  Organ-System: Liver, Stomach

Stimulants or Herbs That Warm the Interior and Expel Cold

These herbs treat Cold lodged in the interior of the body either from a pathogenic influence that has penetrated the organs or from deficiency of Yang. The symptoms can be aversion to cold, cold hands and feet, loose stools, or lack of Qi-energy.

The main Phases of these herbs are Air, Space to dry dampness associated with this pattern and Fire for warming.

These herbs calm Vata and Kapha and aggravate Pitta.

- **Anise Seed—Pimpinella anisum, seed**
  Functional Principle: acrid, warm
  Organ-System: Stomach, Liver, Metabolic, Kidney

- **Bayberry—Myrica cerifera, bark**
  Functional Principle: acrid, astringent, warm
  Organ-System: Metabolic, Lungs, Liver

- **Black Pepper—Piper nigrum, fruit, *hu jiao***
  Functional Principle: acrid, hot
  Organ-System: Large Intestine, Stomach

- **Cayenne Pepper—Capsicum frutescens, fruit**
  Functional Principle: acrid, hot
  Organ-System: Kidneys, Metabolic, Stomach

- **Cinnamon Bark—Cinnamomum cassia, bark, *rou gui***
  Functional Principle: acrid, sweet, hot
  Organ-System: Heart, Kidneys, Liver, Metabolic

- **Cloves—Caryophyllus aromaticus, flower, *ding xiang***
  Functional Principle: acrid, warm
  Organ-System: k, Metabolic, Stomach

- **Fennel Seed—Foeniculum vulgare, fruit, *xiao hui xiang***
  Functional Principle: acrid, warm
  Organ-System: Liver, Kidneys, Metabolic, Stomach

Notes

- **Ginger, dry—Zingiber officinale, dried rhizome, *gan jiang***
  Functional Principle: acrid, hot
  Organ-System: Heart, Lungs, Metabolic, Stomach

- **Horseradish—Amoracia rusticana, root**
  Functional Principle: acrid, hot
  Organ-System: Lungs, Large Intestine, Kidneys

- **Prickly Ash—Zanthoxylum americanum, bark**
  Functional Principle: acrid, warm, diffusing
  Organ-System: Metabolic, Stomach, Kidneys

- **Star Anise—Illicium verum, fruit**
  Functional Principle: acrid, warm
  Organ-System: Stomach, Metabolic, Kidneys

Carminatives or Aromatic Herbs That Transform Dampness

The main pattern here is poor digestion with bloating and distention, poor appetite, little thirst, nausea, and a thick coat on the tongue.

The main Phases of these herbs are Air and Space to dry the dampness and Fire to warm, dry and revive the digestion.

These herbs calm Vata and Kapha.

- **Caraway—Carum carvi, seed**
  Functional Principle: acrid, warm
  Organ-System: Stomach, Large Intestine, Lungs

- **Cardamom—Amomum kravanh, fruit, *bai dou kou***
  Functional Principle: acrid, warm, aromatic
  Organ-System: Lungs, Metabolic, Stomach

- **Cumin—Cuminum cyminum, seed**
  Functional Principle: acrid, cool
  Organ-System: Liver, Metabolic

- **Galangal Seeds—Alpinia katsucadai, seed, *cao dou kou***
  Functional Principle: acrid, warm, aromatic
  Organ-System: Metabolic, Stomach

- **Magnolia Bark—Magnolia officinalis, bark, *hou po***
  Functional Principle: bitter, acrid, warm, aromatic
  Organ-System: Large Intestine, Lungs, Metabolic, Stomach

Notes

- **Patchouli—Agastache rugosa, aerial part, *huo xiang***
  Functional Principle: acrid, warm
  Organ-System: Lungs, Metabolic, Stomach

Digestants or Herbs That Regulate the Qi

These herbs unblock stuck Qi/energy in the body usually of the Stomach and Metabolic-Systems, the Liver-System, or the Lungs-System.

The herbs in this category have the Phases of Air and Space to move stagnation. Some of the herbs have the Fire Phase to dry dampness.

These herbs calm Pitta.

- **Chive—Allium macrostemon, bulb, *xie bai***
  Functional Principle: acrid, bitter, warm
  Organ-System: Large Intestine, Lungs, Stomach

- **Nut Grass—Cyperus rotundus, rhizome, *xiang fu***
  Functional Principle: acrid, bitter, sweet, neutral
  Organ-System: Liver, Triple Burner

- **Rose Petals—Rosa rugosa, flower, *mei gui hua***
  Functional Principle: sweet, bitter, warm
  Organ-System: Liver, Metabolic

- **Sandalwood—Santalum albus, wood, *tan xiang***
  Functional Principle: acrid, warm
  Organ-System: Metabolic, Stomach

- **Tangerine Peel—Citrus reticulata, rind, *chen pi***
  Functional Principle: acrid, bitter, warm, aromatic
  Organ-System: Lungs, Metabolic, Stomach

Herbs That Relieve Food Stagnation

These herbs move stagnation and guide out accumulation caused by improper eating or emotional issues. These herbs can be warm or cooling depending on the condition. Warm conditions can present with bad breath, yellow tongue coat, or abdominal distention. Cool conditions can present with nausea, poor digestion, or white tongue coat.

The main Phases of this category are Earth and Water which have a downward moving action.

These herbs calm Pitta and Kapha.

Notes

- **Barley Sprout—Hordeum vulgare, fruit, *cai ya***
  Functional Principle: sweet, neutral
  Organ-System: Liver, Metabolic, Stomach

- **Hawthorn Berry—Crataegus spp., fruit, *shan zha***
  Functional Principle: sour, sweet, warm
  Organ-System: Liver, Metabolic, Stomach

- **Radish Seed—Raphanus sativus, seed, *lai fu zi***
  Functional Principle: acrid, sweet, neutral
  Organ-System: Lungs, Metabolic, Stomach

- **Rice Sprout—Oryza sativa, fruit, *gu ya***
  Functional Principle: sweet, neutral
  Organ-System: Metabolic, Stomach

Herbs That Regulate the Blood

There are two categories for regulating the Blood: Hemostatics that stop bleeding and herbs that invigorate the Blood or move Blood.

Hemostatics or Herbs That Stop Bleeding

These herbs are used to stop bleeding such as nosebleeds, excessive menstruation, uterine bleeding, bleeding due to trauma, coughing blood, blood in the stool, or blood in the urine. These herbs are not used in a condition of excess Heat causing bleeding.

The main Phases of this category are Space, Air, and Earth for its constricting effect. These herbs calm Pitta and Kapha.

- **Agrimony—Agrimonia pilosa, aerial part**
  Functional Principle: bitter, acrid, neutral
  Organ-System: Lungs, Liver, Metabolic

- **Burnet—Sanguisorba officinalis, root, *di yu***
  Functional Principle: bitter, sour, cold
  Organ-System: Liver, Large Intestine, Stomach

- **Madder Root—Rubia cordifolia, root, *qian cao gen***
  Functional Principle: bitter, cold
  Organ-System: Heart, Liver

- **Mugwort—Artemisia argyi, leaf, *ai ye***
  Functional Principle: bitter, acrid, warm
  Organ-System: Metabolic, Liver, Kidneys

Notes

- **Raspberry Leaves—Rubus chingii, leaf**
  Functional Principle: bitter, cool
  Organ-System: Metabolic, Liver, Kidneys

- **Shepherd's Purse—Capsella bursa-pastoris, whole plant**
  Functional Principle: pungent, sweet, neutral
  Organ-System: Liver, Stomach

- **Thistles—Cirsium japonicum, herb and root, *da ji***
  Functional Principle: sweet, cool
  Organ-System: Liver, Metabolic

Emmenagogues or Herbs That Invigorate the Blood

These herbs are used to treat Blood stasis in different areas of the body. These can be used to treat pain from Blood stasis wherever it may present.

The main Phases of this category are Air and Space for the moving quality and Earth for its nourishing quality.

These herbs increase Kapha.

- **Blue Cohosh—Caulophyllum thalictroides, root**
  Functional Principle: acrid, bitter, warm
  Organ-System: Liver, Lungs

- **Curcuma—Curcuma longa, tuber, *yu jin***
  Functional Principle: acrid, bitter, cool
  Organ-System: Heart, Lungs, Liver

- **Calendula—Calendula officinalis, flower**
  Functional Principle: acrid, bitter, neutral
  Organ-System: Liver, Heart, Lungs

- **Collinsonia—Collinsonia canadensis, root**
  Functional Principle: acrid, sour, warm
  Organ-System: Liver, Pericardium, Lungs, Large Intestine

- **Frankincense—Boswellia carterii, gum, *ru xiang***
  Functional Principle: acrid, bitter, warm
  Organ-System: Heart, Liver, Metabolic

- **Lovage—Ligusticum chuanxiong, root, *chuan xiong***
  Functional Principle: acrid, warm
  Organ-System: Liver, Gall Bladder, Pericardium

Notes

- **Motherwort—Leonorus cardiac, aerial part, *yi mu cao***
  Functional Principle: acrid, bitter, cold
  Organ-System: Heart, Liver, Bladder

- **Myrrh—Comniphora myrrha, resin, *mo yao***
  Functional Principle: bitter, neutral
  Organ-System: Heart, Liver, Metabolic

- **Peach Kernel—Prunus persica, seed, *tao ren***
  Functional Principle: bitter, sweet, neutral
  Organ-System: Heart, Large Intestine, Liver, Lungs

- **Peony, Red—Paeonia veitchii, root, *chi shao***
  Functional Principle: sour, bitter, cold
  Organ-System: Liver, Metabolic

- **Pennyroyal—Hedeoma pulegiodes, aerial part**
  Functional Principle: acrid, bitter, warm
  Organ-System: Liver, Lungs

- **Rose—Rosa rugosa, flower, fruit, *yue ji hua***
  Functional Principle: sweet, warm
  Organ-System: Liver

- **Rue—Ruta graveolens, aerial part**
  Functional Principle: bitter, pungent, warm
  Organ-System: Liver, Metabolic, kidney

- **Safflower—Carthamus tinctorius, flower, *hong hua***
  Functional Principle: acrid, warm
  Organ-System: Heart, Liver

- **Sage—Salvia Miltiorrhiza, root, *dan shen***
  Functional Principle: bitter, cold
  Organ-System: Heart, Pericardium, Liver

- **Tansy—Tanacetum vulgare, flower**
  Functional Principle: bitter, acrid, warm
  Organ-System: Liver, Pericardium

- **Vervain—Verbena officinalis, aerial part**
  Functional Principle: cold, bitter
  Organ-System: Liver, Metabolic

Tonics or Herbs That Tonify

Notes

Herbs that provide tonification will strengthen a body process that is deficient whether it is the Qi/energy, Blood, Yin, or Yang aspect. Each aspect will be discussed separately since the herbs may be different. Yang tonics should be used with caution and only when the practitioner is sure that it is the Yang (associated with adrenal function) that needs to be addressed and not the Yin. If Yang tonics are used when there is Yin deficiency the person's condition will deteriorate.

Tonics—Herbs That Tonify the Qi

These herbs are used to increase energy or Qi in an organ-system especially the Metabolic-System and the Lungs-System.

The main Phases of this category are Water and Earth for their nourishing qualities.

- **American Ginseng—Panax quinquefolium, root, *xi yang shen***
  Functional Principle: sweet, bitter, cold
  Organ-System: Heart, Kidneys, Lungs

- **Astragalus—Astragalus membranaceus, root, *huang qi***
  Functional Principle: sweet, warm
  Organ-System: Lungs, Metabolic

- **Elecampane—Inula japonica, root, *tu mu xiang***
  Functional Principle: sweet, acrid, bitter, warm
  Organ-System: Lungs, Liver, Metabolic

- **Ginseng—Panax ginseng, root, *ren shen***
  Functional Principle: sweet, bitter, warm
  Organ-System: Metabolic, Lungs, Heart

- **Licorice—Glycyrrhiza glabra, root, *gan cao***
  Functional Principle: sweet, neutral
  Organ-System: all

- **Spikenard—Aralia racemosa, root**
  Functional Principle: sweet, acrid, warm
  Organ-System: Lungs, Metabolic

- **Siberian Ginseng—Eleutherococcus senticosus, root and stem, *ci wu jia***
  Functional Principle: acrid, sweet, bitter, warm
  Organ-System: Liver, Kidneys

- **Solomon Seal—Polygonatum sibiricum, rhizome, *huang jing***
  Functional Principle: sweet, neutral
  Organ-System: Kidneys, Lungs, Metabolic

Notes

Tonics—Herbs That Tonify the Blood

These herbs strengthen the Blood. The associated symptoms are pale face, lips, and tongue, Heart palpitations, dry hair, skin, and nails, or irregular menstruation. There may or may not be anemia with Blood deficiency patterns.

The main Phases of this category are Earth and Water for their nourishing and moistening effects.

- **Angelica sinensis, root, *dang gui***
  Functional Principle: sweet, acrid, bitter, warm
  Organ-System: Heart, Liver, Metabolic

- **Lycii berries—Lycium chinensis, fruit, *gou qi zi***
  Functional Principle: sweet, neutral
  Organ-System: Kidneys, Liver

Tonics—Herbs That Tonify Yang

These herbs are used for deficient Yang symptoms such as exhaustion, aversion to cold, sore and achy lower back, and a pale tongue.

The main Phases of this category are Water and Earth for their nourishing properties, with smaller amounts of Space, Air, and Fire for their moving and warming qualities. If the practitioner is going to increase Qi/energy in the system, it must be made to move, or it will result in stagnation and pain.

- **Ashwagandha—Withania somnifera, root**
  Functional Principle: bitter, sweet, warm
  Organ-System: Lungs, Kidneys

- **Astragalus Seed—Astragalus complanatus, seed, *sha yuan ji li***
  Functional Principle: sweet, warm
  Organ-System: Kidneys, Liver

- **Cardamom, Black—Alpinia oxyphylla, fruit, *yi zhi ren***
  Functional Principle: acrid, warm
  Organ-System: Kidneys, Metabolic

- **Damiana—Turnera aphrodisiaca, leaf**
  Functional Principle: acrid, warm
  Organ-System: Kidneys

- **Dodder Seed—Cuscuta chinensis, seed, *tu si zi***
  Functional Principle: acrid, sweet, neutral
  Organ-System: Kidneys, Liver

- **Epimedium—Epimedium grandiflorum, aerial part, *yin yang huo***
  Functional Principle: acrid, sweet, warm
  Organ-System: Kidneys, Liver

- **False Unicorn root—Chamaelirium luteum, root**
  Functional Principle: bitter, warm
  Organ-System: Kidneys, Metabolic

- **Fenugreek seeds—Trigonella foenum-graecum, seed, *hu lu ba***
  Functional Principle: bitter, warm
  Organ-System: Liver, Kidneys

- **Leek Seeds—Allium tuberosum, seed, *jiu zi***
  Functional Principle: acrid, sweet, warm
  Organ-System: Kidneys, Liver

- **Saw Palmetto—Sabal serrulata, fruit**
  Functional Principle: pungent, sweet, warm
  Organ-System: Kidneys, Metabolic, Liver

- **Walnut—Juglans regia, seed, *hu tao ren***
  Functional Principle: sweet, warm
  Organ-System: Kidneys, Large Intestine, Lungs

Tonics—Herbs That Tonify Yin

These herbs are used to nourish and moisten and by moistening they also have cooling properties. The symptoms will be Dryness of the Kidney, Liver, Lungs, Stomach or Intestinal Systems. The Yin of the Heart-System is dealt with under Herbs that Calm the Spirit.

Yin tonics are cooling, sweet, and cloying and can be difficult to digest if there is deficiency of the Metabolic-System. Therefore, they are often combined with herbs that help to digest them.

Yin tonics are mainly Water and Earth Phases.

- **American Ginseng—Panax quinquefolium, root, *xi yang shen***
  Functional Principle: sweet, bitter, cold
  Organ-System: Heart, Kidneys, Lungs

- **Asparagus root—Asparagus cochinchinensis, tuber, *tian men dong***
  Functional Principle: sweet, bitter, cold
  Organ-System: Kidneys, Lungs

- **Devil's Club—Oplopanax horridus, root bark**
  Functional Principle: acrid, bitter, cool
  Organ-System: Metabolic, Lungs

Notes

Notes

- **Lily—Lilium brownie, bulb, *bai he***
  Functional Principle: sweet, bitter, cold
  Organ-System: Heart, Lungs

- **Marshmallow root—Althea officinalis, root**
  Functional Principle: sweet, bitter, cool
  Organ-System: Lungs, Stomach, Kidneys

- **Sesame, Black—Sesamum indicum, seed, *hei zhi ma***
  Functional Principle: sweet, neutral
  Organ-System: Kidneys, Liver

- **Slippery Elm—Ulmus fulva, inner bark**
  Functional Principle: sweet, neutral
  Organ-System: Lungs, Stomach

- **Solomon Seal—Polygonatum sibiricum, rhizome, *yu zhu***
  Functional Principle: sweet, cold
  Organ-System: Lungs, Stomach

Astringents or Herbs That Stabilize and Bind

These herbs are used for excessive urination or excessive sweating. They can also be used to prevent or correct prolapse conditions. The cause of these conditions is usually deficiency within the Metabolic-System whose responsibility is to provide uplift in the body among other things.

The main Phases of these herbs are Earth for its contracting and drying qualities and Space. These two Phases make up the Astringent Taste.

These herbs aggravate Vata.

- **Amaranth—Amaranthus hypochondriacus, aerial part**
  Functional Principle: sweet, neutral
  Organ-System: Metabolic, Kidneys

- **Bistort—Bistorta officinalis, root**
  Functional Principle: astringent, bitter, cool
  Organ-System: Liver, Small Intestine, Large Intestine

- **Blackberry—Rubus spp., leaf, root bark**
  Functional Principle: bitter, astringent, neutral
  Organ-System: Stomach, Small Intestine, Large Intestine

- **Cranesbill—Geranium spp., root**
  Functional Principle: astringent, bitter, neutral
  Organ-System: Stomach, intestines, Liver, Heart

- **Ephedra Root—Ephedra spp., root, *ma huang***
  Functional Principle: sweet, neutral
  Organ-System: Lungs

- **Eyebright—Euphrasia officinalis, whole plant**
  Functional Principle: bitter, mildly astringent, cool
  Organ-System: Liver, Lungs

- **Ginkgo—Ginkgo biloba, seed, *bai guo***
  Functional Principle: sweet, bitter, astringent, neutral
  Organ-System: Kidneys, Lungs

- **Horse Chestnut—Aesculus hippocastanum, seed, bark**
  Functional Principle: bitter, astringent, neutral, toxic
  Organ-System: Metabolic, Lungs

- **Lady's Mantle—Alchemilla vulgaris, whole plant**
  Functional Principle: bitter, astringent, neutral
  Organ-System: Metabolic, Kidneys

- **Nettles—Urtica dioica, leaf**
  Functional Principle: bland, bitter, cool
  Organ-System: Small Intestine, Bladder, Lungs

- **Nutmeg—Myristica fragrans, seed, *rou dou kou***
  Functional Principle: acrid, warm
  Organ-System: Large Intestine, Metabolic, Stomach

- **Oak—Quercus alba, bark, fruit**
  Functional Principle: astringent, bitter, neutral
  Organ-System: Metabolic, Stomach, Small Intestine, Large Intestine

- **Pomegranate—Punica granatum, rind, *shi liu pi***
  Functional Principle: sour, astringent, warm
  Organ-System: Kidneys, Large Intestine, Stomach

- **Raspberry—Rubus chingii, fruit, *fu pen zi***
  Functional Principle: sweet, astringent, warm
  Organ-System: Kidneys, Liver

- **Rose Hips—Rosa rugosa, fruit, *jin ying zi***
  Functional Principle: sour, astringent, neutral
  Organ-System: Bladder, Kidneys, Large Intestine

Notes

Notes

- **Schisandra—Schisandra sinensis, fruit, *wu wei zi***
  Functional Principle: sour, warm
  Organ-System: Heart, Kidneys, Lungs

- **Sumac—Rhus chinensis, gallnut, *wu bei zi***
  Functional Principle: sour, salty, cold
  Organ-System: Kidneys, Large Intestine, Lungs

- **Witch Hazel—Hamemelis virginiana, leaf, bark**
  Functional Principle: bitter, astringent, neutral
  Organ-System: Heart, Stomach, intestines

- **Yerba Mansa—Anemopsis californica, leaf, root**
  Functional Principle: bitter, astringent, warm
  Organ-System: Lungs, Metabolic

Nervines or Herbs That Calm the Spirit

These herbs treat the nervous system that can manifest with symptoms of insomnia, Heart palpitations, and anxiety. There are three categories—Herbs that Sedate and Calm the Spirit, Cooling or Warming Herbs that Nourish the Heart and Calm the Spirit and Aromatic Herbs that Open the Orifices.

Substances That Anchor, Settle, and Calm the Spirit

These are minerals chosen for their weight and density to anchor the Spirit.

The main Phases are Water and Earth for the heaviness.

These herbs calm Vata and aggravate Kapha.

- **Amber—resin, *hu po***
  Functional Principle: sweet, neutral
  Organ-System: Bladder, Heart, Liver

- **Dragon Bone—*long gu***
  Functional Principle: sweet, astringent, neutral
  Organ-System: Heart, Kidneys, Liver

- **Hematite—Haematitum, *dai zhe shi***
  Functional Principle: bitter, cold
  Organ-System: Heart, Liver, Pericardium

- **Magnetite—Magnetitum, *ci shi***
  Functional Principle: acrid, salty, cold
  Organ-System: Kidneys, Liver

- **Oyster Shell—Ostrea gigas, shell, *mu li***
  Functional Principle: salty, astringent, cool
  Organ-System: Liver, Kidneys

Notes

Cooling Herbs That Nourish the Heart and Calm the Spirit

These herbs calm the Heart-System by cooling the uprising heat usually due to stress. Some symptoms would be insomnia, especially between 1-3a.m., and sudden panic with Heart palpitations. These herbs may need to be combined with others that are Sweet to further strengthen the Heart-System.

The main Phases are Earth for its grounding and nourishing qualities and Space and Air for their cooling effect.

These herbs calm Vata.

- **Arbor-Vitae—Biota orientalis, seed, *bai zi ren***
  Functional Principle: sweet, neutral
  Organ-System: Heart, Kidneys, Large Intestine, Metabolic

- **California Poppy—Eschscholzia californica, aerial part**
  Functional Principle: bitter, cool
  Organ-System: Liver, Heart

- **Chamomile—Matricaria chamomilla, Anthemis nobilis, flower**
  Functional Principle: bitter, acrid, neutral
  Organ-System: Liver, Stomach, Lungs

- **Hops—Humulus lupulus, strobili**
  Functional Principle: bitter, cool
  Organ-System: Heart, Liver

- **Lady's Slipper—Cypripedium acaule, root**
  Functional Principle: acrid, sweet, neutral
  Organ-System: Liver, Heart

- **Passion Flower—Passiflora incarnata, aerial part**
  Functional Principle: bitter, cool
  Organ-System: Heart, Liver

- **Scullcap—Scutellaria lateriflora, whole plant**
  Functional Principle: bitter, cool
  Organ-System: Heart, Liver

- **Wood Betony—Betonica officinalis, whole plant**
  Functional Principle: bitter, cool
  Organ-System: Liver, Heart

Notes

Warming Herbs That Nourish the Heart and Calm the Spirit

These herbs are for nervous systems that present with the condition of Cold.

The main Phases are Air, Space, and Fire.

These herbs calm Vata.

- **Kava—Piper methysticum, rhizome**
  Functional Principle: pungent, bitter, warm
  Organ-System: Bladder, Kidneys, intestines

- **Valerian—Valeriana officinalis, root**
  Functional Principle: acrid, bitter, warm
  Organ-System: Liver, Heart

Aromatic Herbs That Open the Orifices

These herbs are used to unblock the senses and revive the nervous system. These herbs have a strong dispersing action to clear and restore the senses bringing a stronger and clearer consciousness. They can be used with symptoms of seizures, clouded consciousness, and stroke. These can be hot or cold conditions.

The main Phases in this category are Air and Space for their dispersing qualities and Fire for its penetrating quality.

These herbs calm Kapha.

- **Bay—Laurus nobilis, leaf**
  Functional Principle: acrid, warm
  Organ-System: Heart, Metabolic

- **Benzoinum—Styrax benzoin, resin, *an xi xiang***
  Functional Principle: acrid, bitter, neutral
  Organ-System: Heart, Liver, Metabolic

- **Calamus—Acorus calamus, rhizome, *shi chang pu***
  Functional Principle: acrid, warm, aromatic
  Organ-System: Heart, Stomach

Antispasmodics or Herbs That Extinguish Wind and Stop Tremors

Wind is a pathogenic factor that can create tremors, spasms and tics. Wind most often affects the Liver-System with Wind-Heat creating headaches, blurry vision, tinnitus, Heart palpitations, twitches, and irritability. If this pattern continues it can result in tremors, facial paralysis, and aphasia.

The Phases of this category are Water, Fire, Space, and Air.
These herbs calm Vata.

Notes

- **Abalone Shell—Haliotis diversicolor, shell, *shi jue ming***
  Functional Principle: salty, cold
  Organ-System: Kidneys, Liver

- **Blackhaw—Viburnum prunifolium, root bark**
  Functional Principle: bitter, cool
  Organ-System: Liver

- **Caltrop—Tribulus terrestris, fruit, *bai ji li***
  Functional Principle: acrid, bitter, warm
  Organ-System: Liver, Lungs

- **Cramp Bark—Viburnum opulus, branch bark**
  Functional Principle: bitter, cool
  Organ-System: Liver, Heart, Lungs, Bladder

- **Gastrodia—Gastrodia elata, rhizome, *tian ma***
  Functional Principle: sweet, neutral
  Organ-System: Liver

- **Lobelia—Lobelia inflata, leaf, flower, seed**
  Functional Principle: bitter, neutral
  Organ-System: Liver, Lungs, Heart, Small Intestine

- **Uncaria—Uncaria sinensis, twig, *gou teng***
  Functional Principle: sweet, cool
  Organ-System: Heart, Liver

Transform Phlegm

Phlegm is considered a sticky, toxic substance that can clog or accumulate in any area of the body. The symptoms in the Lungs-System may be coughing, wheezing, and heaviness in the chest; in the Metabolic-System may be nausea, vomiting, poor appetite, distention and coughing. Symptoms in the channels may be goiter or scrofula. Phlegm obstructing the Heart-System can be seizures, trans-ischemic attacks or stroke.

There are cooling and warming categories to these herbs.

These herbs calm Pitta and Kapha.

Cooling Herbs That Transform Phlegm-Heat

These herbs are cold and contain the Phases of Space and Air and Water and Earth all of which have cooling properties.

Notes

- **Bamboo—Bambusa, textilis, concretion, *tian zhu huang***
  Functional Principle: sweet, cool
  Organ-System: Gall Bladder, Heart, Liver

- **Bamboo Sap—Bambusa breviflora, sap, *zhu li***
  Functional Principle: sweet, very cold
  Organ-System: Heart, Lungs, Stomach

- **Clam Shell—Cyclinae sinensis, shell, *hai ge ke***
  Functional Principle: bitter, salty, neutral
  Organ-System: Kidneys, Lungs, Stomach

- **Chickweed—Stellaria dichotoma, whole plant, *yin chai hu***
  Functional Principle: bitter, sweet, cool
  Organ-System: Lungs, Stomach

- **Horehound—Marrubium vulgare, leaf**
  Functional Principle: bitter, cool
  Organ-System: Lungs, Metabolic, Liver, Heart

- **Kelp—Laminaria japonica, thallus, *kun bu***
  Functional Principle: salty, cold
  Organ-System: Kidneys, Liver, Stomach

- **Pumice—*fu hai shi***
  Functional Principle: salty, cold
  Organ-System: Lungs

- **Seaweed—Sargassum palladium, *hai zao***
  Functional Principle: bitter, salty, cold
  Organ-System: Kidneys, Liver, Lungs, Stomach

Warming Herbs That Transform Phlegm-Cold

These herbs are warming and contain the Phases of Air, Space, and Fire.

- **Balloon Flower—Platycodon grandiflorum, root, *jie geng***
  Functional Principle: bitter, acrid, neutral
  Organ-System: Lungs

- **Bloodroot—Sanguinaria canadensis, rhizome**
  Functional Principle: bitter, acrid, hot, toxic
  Organ-System: Lungs, Heart, Liver

Notes

- **Elecampane—Inula japonica, flower, *xuan fu hua***
  Functional Principle: bitter, acrid, warm
  Organ-System: Liver, Lungs, Stomach, Metabolic

- **Eucalyptus—Eucalyptus globulus, leaf**
  Functional Principle: acrid, warm
  Organ-System: Lungs, Kidneys

- **Grindelia—Grindelia spp., flower**
  Functional Principle: bitter, pungent, warm
  Organ-System: Lungs, Kidneys

- **Mustard Seeds—Brassica alba, seed, *bai jie zi***
  Functional Principle: acrid, warm
  Organ-System: Lungs

- **Thyme—Thymus vulgaris, leaf, flower**
  Functional Principle: acrid, warm
  Organ-System: Lungs, Liver, Stomach

- **Yerba Santa—Eriodictyon spp., leaf**
  Functional Principle: acrid, warm
  Organ-System: Lungs, Large Intestine, Stomach

Antitussives or Herbs That Relieve Coughing & Wheezing

See also Expectorant

- **Apricot Seed—Prunus armeniaca, seed, *xing ren***
  Functional Principle: bitter, warm
  Organ-System: Large Intestine, Lungs

- **Aster—Aster tataricus, root, *zi wan***
  Functional Principle: bitter, warm
  Organ-System: Lungs

- **Coltsfoot—Tussilago farfara, flower, *kuan dong hua***
  Functional Principle: acrid, warm
  Organ-System: Lungs

- **Lungwort—Pulmonaria officinalis, whole plant**
  Functional Principle: astringent, sweet, bitter, cool
  Organ-System: Lungs, Stomach

Notes

- **Mulberry—Morus alba, bark, *sang bai pi***
  Functional Principle: sweet, cold
  Organ-System: Lungs, Metabolic

- **Mullein—Verbascum thapsus, leaf, flower**
  Functional Principle: bitter, astringent, cool
  Organ-System: Lungs, Stomach

- **Wild Cherry Bark—Prunus virginiana, bark**
  Functional Principle: acrid, astringent, warm
  Organ-System: Metabolic, Lungs

Parasiticides

The herbs in this category are to be used for short periods of time as they can be depleting to the body.

They will aggravate Vata.

- **Betel Nut—Areca catechu, seed, *bing lang***
  Functional Principle: acrid, biter, warm
  Organ-System: Large Intestine, Stomach

- **Elm—Ulmus macrocarpus, prepared fruit, *wu yi***
  Functional Principle: bitter, cold
  Organ-System: Large Intestine, Stomach

- **Garlic—Allium sativum, bulb, *da suan***
  Functional Principle: acrid, warm
  Organ-System: Large Intestine, Lungs, Metabolic, Stomach

- **Male Fern—Dryopteris crassirhizoma, rhizome, *guan zhong***
  Functional Principle: bitter, cold
  Organ-System: Liver, Metabolic

- **Pinkroot—Spigelia marylandica, herb**
  Functional Principle: bitter, acrid, cold
  Organ-System: Large Intestine, Stomach

- **Pomegranate—Punica granatum, rind, *shi liu pi***
  Functional Principle: sour, astringent, warm
  Organ-System: Kidneys, Large Intestine, Stomach

- **Pumpkin Seeds—Curcubita moschata, seed, *nan gua zi***
  Functional Principle: sweet, neutral
  Organ-System: Large Intestine, Stomach

Part Four:

Future Systems Medicine

Notes

Chapter 15:

Cosmology of Herbal Medicine

The cosmos is an organized and harmonious system governed by Nature's laws that are the same throughout our universe. Even if you are on another continent or planet, the laws controlling the actions of matter-energy and, specifically plants, herbs, and food, are the same. Therefore, the following chart is a synthesis of herbal medicine based on the information in the foregoing chapters.

If you can determine the Tastes of an herb, the *Cosmology of Herbal Medicine* chart will give you the Phases, the actions of the Tastes, and the general conditions it will treat according to Ayurveda and Chinese Medicine providing you understand The Functional Principles of Eastern medicine.

You can read the chart from left to right by first determining the Taste and Phases; or you can read the chart from right to left and, by knowing the person's condition according to Ayurveda or Chinese Medicine, the chart will tell you the strategy of the Functional Principle needed and directs you to the Taste of the herbs needed.

The chart is *not* to be used by plugging in a Taste or condition as in an equation—that would be linear thinking, but as a guide to help the student herbalist learn systems herbal medicine.

A Note About Food and Taste

In order to discern the tastes of an herb, food, or any substance, one must have a clear palate. That means one must have a balanced and healthy (for your doshas) diet and lifestyle that includes all Six Tastes, in moderation, in order to differentiate The Six Tastes accurately.

Dr. Robert Svoboda, Ayurvedic physician, states, ". . . the main factor that makes for disease is the indulgence in unwholesome diet." He adds, "The fundamental cause for all

Notes

ama, or toxins—the source of disease, is indigestible desire." Desire can be in the form of unwholesome foods we have been accustomed to eat.[1]

Michael Greger, M.D., in his book *How Not to Die,* provides substantial evidence that a whole food, plant-based diet is the best way to avoid disease, even sub-clinical disease patterns that damage our ability to accurately perceive and interpret our world.[2]

This conclusion is corroborated in Chinese Medicine which asserts that most mental symptoms are due to *phlegm, ama* or toxins that obstruct the system of the Heart-Mind or *shen.* The source of these toxins is unwholesome foods, such as processed foods and the greasy, slimy, and energetically hot animal products to which people have become habituated. (Refer to Chapter 6—The Six Tastes) These patterns of disharmony in the Heart-Mind-System can lead to symptoms of manic-depression, violent behavior, confusion, and lethargy.

Therefore, if we choose a high-protein animal-based diet, our body-minds become toxic, stagnant, dull, and confused. Consequently, one will not be able to discern The Six Tastes accurately enough to determine which of The Six Tastes are present in an herb or food.

Eastern medicine extrapolates further and observes how our societies have been distorted by the unwholesome foods we have been eating. Just as a computer can give output based only on the quality of information it is given, our minds can make decisions only based on the quality of input it is given. Thus, the old adage of "garbage in—garbage out," or unwholesome food in—unwholesome decisions out. In Ayurveda we say "food is medicine"; or if not properly digested, which unwholesome food never is, it is considered a poison.

Think of an ecological system where a chemical poison has been introduced or a minor component has been eliminated and how that system begins to break down, and you begin to see the parallels between the macrocosmic environment and the microcosmic human body.

Table–15-1

COSMOLOGY OF HERBAL MEDICINE

TASTE & PHASES	FUNCTIONAL PRINCIPLES	AYURVEDA	CHINESE MEDICINE
BITTER Space & Air	Decreases Heat Cooling & Drying	Reduces Pitta & Kapha Increases Vata	Decreases Yang Decreases Yin
PUNGENT Air & Fire	Increases Digestive Fire Drying & Heating	Reduces Kapha Increases Vata & Pitta	Increases Yang Decreases Yin
SOUR Fire & Earth	Increases Metabolism Heating & Moistening	Reduces Vata Increases Pitta & Kapha	Increases Yang Increases Yin
ASTRINGENT Air & Earth	Decreases Water Cooling & Drying	Reduces Pitta & Kapha Increases Vata	Decreases Yang Decreases Yin
SALTY Fire & Water	Increases Water Heating & Moistening	Reduces Vata Increases Pitta & Kapha	Increases Yang Increases Yin
SWEET Water & Earth	Nutritive Moistening & Cooling	Reduces Vata & Pitta Increases Kapha	Decreases Yang Increases Yin

Notes

Chapter 16:

Back to the Future: Systems Medicine

No attempts to refine our present medical system will prove ultimately successful unless they address the deficiencies of the most basic assumptions on which the system rests.

—Larry Dossey, M.D.[1]

According to quantum physics, it is impossible to precisely determine, simultaneously, the exact location and the velocity of a moving object because any attempt at measurement of either inevitably involves change in the other.[2]

The same paradox exists when analyzing living cells. One must kill the cell, forever changing it in order to analyze it. While all the chemical constituents are present, the relationships in and between the cell structures are lost, forever changing what it once was. Its function and therefore its inherent value are lost.

All modern medicines are based on the analysis of dead cells and dead organisms. Therefore, the interrelationships determining the function of the networks between cells and organs will always elude the medical researcher or doctor. Consequently, one must resort to metaphor or poetry to appreciate the value of the relationships between living cells and the various systems of the living body. The physicist Niels Bohr (1885-1962) also suggested that many of the new concepts from modern physics could best be described metaphorically, and more accurately, in the language of poetry.[3] It is why Eastern medicine has always used the poetry of nature, such as The Five Phases, to describe the ecology of the living body.

The functions of the various organ-systems of the body are more involved and interrelated than modern medicine, with its limited mechanistic presumptions, understands. The liver, for example, has far more influence and interrelationships in the body than just a blood purifier; and blood test numbers give us limited information about the ecology of

Notes

the entire Liver-System; it only tells us what may be happening at the moment the blood was taken. Modern medicine has a responsibility to stop relying on measurements, begin to perceive and respect their patients and recognize the patterns between the systems of their patient's body as a whole.

Modern medicine is attempting to correct their approach of disease management and "sick care." It has recognized that modern medicine is fragmented and ineffective for chronic conditions; that it is reactive healthcare based on limited and objective measurements; measurements that overwhelm the physicians with data without providing a definitive method of how to accurately qualify the data. The physicians then often over-react, as opposed to respond, which puts their patients at risk. This can be observed when a patient is given one more powerful drug after another and continues to not respond.

Physicist, Amit Goswami states,

> *Once you see consciousness as the ground of all being, it is hard to carry on the often meaningless, materialist research programs that form the bulk of the academic, governmental, and industrial research.*[4]

However, most modern medicine continues to manage chronic diseases for which it was never designed. Its original design (See Chapter 3) was mechanistic heroic medicine—finding and fixing what is broken, such as surgery and dialysis or saving lives subsequent to accidents. In its earlier days, heroic medicine, on which modern medicine was built, is what we now consider as barbaric, such as bloodletting and purging. Heroic medicine examples today are cardiopulmonary resuscitation and the use of multiple drugs to maintain blood pressure.

Amit Goswami, physicist says,

> *Some of these material-realist doctrines, such as objectivity, determinism, and epiphenomenalism, fly in the face of our common sense. . . . We must give up habitual acceptance of the material-realist doctrines because, frankly, quantum mechanics has proven some of them to be outright wrong and has cast grave doubt on the validity of the rest.*[5]

The wheel has already been invented. It is time to investigate systems-medicine that have worked for thousands of years in order to rebuild a new system on a solid and proven foundation. We need a new map for medicine based on the new (now over 100 years old) information and insights that have come to us from modern physics and from ancient Eastern medicine. Ayurveda and Chinese Medicine are proven to be true health-promoting modalities that continue to remain viable and effective healthcare systems.

Health is the Music

Health is more than the sum of your mere body parts and processes; it is an indivisible whole that includes your emotions and consciousness. According to Ayurveda, Chinese Medicine, *and* modern physics, you are essentially dynamic processes and patterns that

Notes

are fundamental to who you are that would be lost and meaningless if viewed as separate parts. By believing laboratory tests provide an indication of health is to assume that reading random, isolated, and individual musical notes will tell you what symphony is playing. And, if we try to change the inherent notes with foreign substances (drugs), we lose the harmony in the body-mind symphony.

Physician Larry Dossey, M.D. in his profound book, *Space, Time and Medicine*, states,

> *An expanded view of consciousness [according to modern physics] leads us to the conclusion that there is no such thing as a physical examination, and the error of the patient who thinks he is getting one is exceeded, perhaps, only by that of the physician who believes he is performing one.*[6]

Health comes from how you compose the musical notes of your life; from what you eat and what you do to what you think—*YOU* are the conductor of your orchestra creating your own unique symphony. Health is not in the notes; health is the music!

Into the Future

The mechanistic modern medical model must change. To do that, it needs to change how its physicians *think* in order to change the way it works. Modern medicine needs to change its mechanics-physicians into "Systems-Physicians;" nothing else will be adequate to make modern medicine into a sustainable true healthcare system.

If a medical system has lasted as long as Eastern medicine, it is because it continues to offer significant benefits that work effectively to heal. Therefore, why not use the systems-thinking of Eastern medicine to train Western medicine practitioners in:

1. **Yin, Yang, and Qi**—to understand and value the inter-relationships and interdependence of organ-systems and tissues in the body and all living things.

   This engenders respect for the person and enables the systems-physician to perceive the person as an individual with a unique perspective, patterns, innate energy/Qi, and therefore, needs. It informs the systems-physician of the complex interrelationships, inter-dependence, and functions of the organ-systems and substances, and the influences of environment so the person could be treated as a unique whole. In addition, the systems-physician would be able to determine the root-cause of the condition and avoid treating symptoms.

2. **The Five Phases**—to understand and value how the basic qualities of natural processes function in the body and nature.

   This helps the systems-physician to more accurately diagnose according to the physiological and pathological relationships among the organ-systems which will lead to the correct treatment strategies, as opposed to diagnosing and treating symptoms.

Notes

3. **The Six Tastes**—to understand the physical effects of The Five Phases on the body and to provide a system of classifying the use of drugs and drug combinations, herbal medicine, and food.

   This enables the systems-physician to counsel the person on specific lifestyle, food guidelines, and herbal medicines to help reverse or moderate their condition. In doing so, the person becomes part of their healing process improving compliance and empowering them. It would also reduce the need for drugs.

   There are experienced Eastern herbal medicine practitioners who already understand the classification of many drugs according to Eastern medicine principles. This would eliminate the guesswork of prescribing drugs, if needed, and provide information on which drug would work best on an individual person and their condition. In most cases, a Systems-Herbalist could use sophisticated herbal medicine instead of drugs.

4. **The Eight Principles**—to provide a system of assessing pathological changes and diagnosis, and determine treatment strategies—how, when, and on whom they should be used.

   This helps the systems-physician define and understand the overall expressions of the patterns of disharmony in the person; to assess pathological changes in the overall body systems, and psychological and emotional traits. Identifying the pattern of disharmony integrates the diagnosis, pathology, and treatment principles.

5. **The Four *Doshas***—to understand and value the pattern of the whole person (context) being treated — physical, mental, spiritual—which in turn, gives further comprehension to the four aspects above.

   Understanding this gives the systems-physician insight to the true nature of a person—body, mind, spirit—and how they would best be treated and counseled.

6. **The Four Observations**—to "see" and inter-relate with the person as opposed to simply reading medical tests and overlooking the person who has the condition.

7. **Tongue and Pulse Assessment**—to provide diagnostic techniques to determine where, how, and the extent of pathogenic factors, and patterns of disharmony.

8. **Learn a regular meditation/introspection practice** to improve focus, memory, mental clarity, and reduce stress.

Once physicians change from linear to systems-thinking, the medical structure itself will change to accommodate the new thinking. Until then the current way the medical structure functions cannot be fixed due to the mechanistic premises it is based on.

Medical doctors would have to be trained to incorporate the new systems-thinking and perhaps have an Eastern medicine Systems Herbalist available with whom they could collaborate. Qualified Eastern herbal practitioners and acupuncturists would be available or would work directly with the systems-physicians in hospitals as they do in China.

Notes

There is also the successful system China inaugurated in the 1960s that trained more than one million people in preventive Eastern medicine treatments combined with basic Western medical care. These service-oriented "Barefoot Doctors" provided primary medical care to their communities with the objective of keeping people healthy. These para-medical physicians provided preventive healthcare with, for example, counseling on nutrition, treatment for common illnesses, and prescriptions for herbal formulas and basic medications. This harmony of Eastern and Western medicine in China has shown how to bring together the positive aspects of each, help to keep medical costs down, and improve the quality of healthcare for all people. Unfortunately, the privatization of Western medicine in China around 1980 brought the Barefoot Doctor program to an end. Subsequently the health-related tragedies of the people substantially increased.[7]

Action to establish the above information would give us the beginnings of a system of genuine healthcare promoting and encouraging health for all, instead of managing disease after it has occurred. We would not be discarding the efficacy of biomedical medicine but enhancing it. There would be far fewer drugs or surgery needed because many conditions could be detected before they become diseases. Modern medicine would be more humane with its focus on maintaining health and quality of life. People would be counseled on lifestyle practices according to their predominantly manifesting and/or out-of-balance *dosha*s (patterns) helping to make them responsible for their health and healing.

Appendix:

New Terminology

Identity—*Ahamkara* in Ayurveda
The ego or consciousness.

Daily Essence = Post-Heaven Essence in Chinese Medicine
The refined substances derived from digestion.

Heart-Mind = Shen in Chinese Medicine
The root of the spirit that includes consciousness, emotions, and thoughts.

Innate Essence = Pre-Heaven Essence in Chinese Medicine
Derived from the parents, it determines our basic constitution, strength, and vitality.

Metabolic-System = Digestive system; Spleen in Chinese Medicine
The organ-system responsible for digestion, assimilation, and transportation of food and Fluids.

Phase = Element
A stage in a series of processes of change.

Original Constitution—*Prakruti* in Ayurveda
The basic constitution, or doshic proportions one inherits at conception.

Perceiver = Duality of Awareness—*Rajas* in Ayurveda
The principles of kinetic energy, activity, emotion, turbulence and discordance.

Notes

Perception = Awareness of Oneness—*Sattva* in Ayurveda
The principles of free-will, potential energy, intelligence and harmony; encompass the higher values and qualities of truth, beauty, goodness, honesty, humility, and compassion.

Perceived = Energy/Matter—*Tamas* in Ayurveda
The principles of inertia, darkness, dullness, and resistance.

Systems Herbalist—An herbalist who is thoroughly trained in systems-thinking Eastern herbal medicine in their clinical practice.

Systems Physician—A medical doctor who has been trained in and uses systems-thinking in their medical practice.

Unbalanced State—*Vikruti* in Ayurveda
The *doshic* balance other than one's original prakruti.

Works Cited

Introduction

1. Dossey. *Space, Time & Medicine*, p 220.
2. Goswami. *The Visionary Window*, p 19.

Chapter 1

1. Paul Dirac as quoted in Dossey. *Space, Time & Medicine*, p 224.
2. "Theory of Relativity."
3. "Introduction to Quantum Mechanics."
4. Capra. *The Tao of Physics*, p 8.
5. Capra. p 69.
6. Capra. p 173.

Chapter 2

1. Capra. *The Tao of Physics*, p 277.
2. Capra. *The Web of Life*, p 122.
3. Manbiot. "How Wolves Change Rivers."
4. Capra. *The Turning Point*, p 123.
5. Tolkien. *The Lord of the Rings*, p 259.
6. Urantia Foundation. *The Urantia Book*, p 141.
7. Capra. *The Turning Point*, p 92.
8. Candice Pert as quoted in Capra. *The Web of Life*, p 282-4.
9. Johnson. "Ninety-Six Words for Love."
10. Dossey. *Space, Time & Medicine*, p 42.
11. Capra. *The Tao of Physics*, p 42.
12. Urantia Foundation. *The Urantia Book*, p 2078.
13. David Bohm as quoted in Dossey. *Space, Time and Medicine*, p 206.
14. Capra. *The Tao of Physics*, p 42.

Chapter 3

1. Bohm. *Wholeness and the Implicate Order,* p 23.
2. Kaptchuk. *The Web That Has No Weaver,* p xx.
3. Capra. *The Web of Life,* p 268.
4. Humberto Maturana and Francisco Varela as quoted in Capra. The Web of Life, p 269.
5. Werner Heisenberg as quoted in Dossey. *Space, Time & Medicine*, p 233.
6. Bohm. *Wholeness and the Implicate Order,* p 19.
7. Ludwig von Bertalanffy as quoted in Capra. *The Web of Life,* p 177.
8. Capra. *The Turning Point*, p 104.
9. Capra. *The Tao of Physics*, p 225.
10. Griggs. *Green Pharmacy,* p 253.
11. Kerr White as quoted in Griggs. *Green Pharmacy*, p 252.
12. Griggs. *Green Pharmacy*, p 253.
13. Capra. *The Web of Life,* p 81.
14. Capra. *The Turning Point*, p 124.
15. Griggs. *Green Pharmacy,* p 330.
16. Urantia Foundation. *The Urantia Book*, p 992.
17. As quoted in Bensky and Barolet. *Chinese Herbal Medicine Formulas & Strategies,* p 5.
18. Capra. *The Tao of Physics*, p 131.
19. Sheldrake. *Science Set Free*, p 46-7.
20. Capra. *The Web of Life,* p 36.
21. Capra. *The Tao of Physics*, p 36.
22. Gobbi. "Pharmacopsychiatry."
23. Remen. "Helping, Fixing or Serving?"

Chapter 4

1. Goswami. *The Visionary Window*, p 228.
2. Green. "Why is it that eating spicy, "hot" food causes the same physical reactions as does physical heat?"
3. Barclay & Donato. p 1.
4. Bensky and Barolet. *Formulas & Strategies,* p 14.
5. Bensky and Barolet. p 16-17.
6. Ibid. p 14.
7. Ibid. p 14.
8. Ibid. p 15.
9. Ibid. p 15.

Chapter 5

1. Capra. *The Tao of Physics*, p 287.
2. Capra. *The Tao of Physics*, p 329.
3. Selbie. *The Physics of God*, p 70-71.

4. Sheldrake. *Science Set Free,* p 99-100.
5. Bohm. *Wholeness and the Implicate Order*, p 53.
6. "What Is the Cloud."

Chapter 6

1. Fred Alan Wolfe as quoted in Goswami. *The Self Aware Universe,* p xiv.
2. Green. "Why is it that eating spicy, "hot" food causes the same physical reactions as does physical heat?"
3. Bensky and Gamble. *Chinese Herbal Medicine Materia Medica*, p 6.
4. Bensky and Gamble. p 6.
5. Sidel. *A Barefoot Doctor's Manual*, p 568.
6. Bensky and Gamble. *Materia Medica,* p xvi.
7. Bensky and Gamble. p 7.
8. Bensky and Gamble. p xvi.
9. Bensky and Gamble. p 6.

Chapter 7

1. Capra. *The Tao of Physics*, p 326.
2. Capra. p 197.
3. Capra. *The Tao of Physics*, p 291.
4. Goswami. *The Self-Aware Universe,* p 188.
5. Capra. *The Tao of Physics,* p 326.
6. Goswami. *The Self-Aware Universe,* p 88.
7. Urantia Foundation. *The Urantia Book*, p 2078.
8. Urantia Foundation. p 482.
9. Capra. *The Tao of Physics*, p 46.
10. Capra. p 68.
11. Urantia Foundation. *The Urantia Book,* p 481.
12. Bohm. *Wholeness and the Implicate Order,* p 142.
13. Lakshmi. *Scientific Basis for Herbal Therapies,* p 21.
14. Frawley and Lad. *Yoga of Herbs*, p 4.
15. Capra. *The Web of Life,* p 178.
16. Frawley and Lad. *The Yoga of Herb,* p 5.
17. Urantia Foundation. *The Urantia Book,* p 483.
18. Capra. *The Tao of Physics*, p 142.
19. Capra. p 141.
20. John Wheeler as quoted in Dossey. *Space, Time, and Medicine*, p 195.
21. Capra. *The Web of Life*, p 140.
22. Capra. p 175.
23. Bohm. *Wholeness and the Implicate Order,* p 11.
24. Ludwig von Bertalanffy as quoted in Capra. *The Web of Life*, p 177.
25. Capra. p 85.
26. Capra. p 193.

27. Capra. p 192.
28. Lad. *Textbook of Ayurveda, Volume I,* p 42
29. Lad. p 43.
30. Lad. p 44.

Chapter 8

1. Capra. *The Tao of Physics,* p 166.
2. Ridley. *Genome,* p 65.
3. Capra. *The Tao of Physics,* p 146.
4. Mastin. "Physics of the Universe."
5. Capra. *The Tao of Physics,* p 225.
6. Bohm. *Wholeness and the Implicate Order,* p 9.
7. Bohm. p 145.
8. Capra. *The Web of Life,* p 37.
9. Eugene Wigner as quoted in Dossey. *Space, Time & Medicine,* p 208.

Chapter 9

1. Dossey. *Space, Time & Medicine,* p 112.

Chapter 10

1. Dossey. *Space, Time & Medicine,* p 84.

Chapter 11

1. Capra. *The Tao of Physics,* p 42.

Chapter 12

1. Bensky and Barolet. *Formulas & Strategies,* p 5.
2. Bensky and Barolet. p 9.
3. Rene Dubois as quoted in Metzner. "The Causes of Disease: The Great Debate."
4. Bensky and Barolet. *Formulas & Strategies,* p 7.
5. Bensky and Barolet. p 8.
6. Bensky and Barolet. p 9.
7. Bensky and Barolet. p 11.
8. Bensky and Barolet. p 10.
9. Bensky and Barolet. p 126.
10. Bensky and Barolet. p 158.
11. Bensky and Barolet. p 10.
12. Bensky and Barolet. p 11.

Chapter 13

1. Svoboda. *Ayurveda. Life, Health, & Longevity*, p 157.
2. Bensky and Gamble. *Materia Medica*, p 66.
3. Capra. *The Turning Point,* p 156.
4. Bensky and Barolet. *Formulas & Strategies,* p 215.

Chapter 14

1. Bensky and Gamble. *Materia Medica*, p 66.
2. Bensky and Gamble. p 115.
3. Bensky and Gamble. p 131.
4. Bensky and Gamble. p 155.

Chapter 15

1. Svoboda. *Ayurveda. Life, Health, & Longevity*, p 161-2.
2. Greger. *How Not to Die*, p 1-14.

Chapter 16

1. Dossey. *Space, Time & Medicine*, p 224.
2. Urantia Foundation. *The Urantia Book*, p 737.
3. Niels Bohr as quoted in Dossey. *Space, Time & Medicine*, p 113.
4. Goswami. *The Visionary Window*, p 75.
5. Goswami. p 29-30.
6. Dossey. *Space, Time & Medicine*, p 210.
7. "Barefoot Doctor."

Bibliography

Ahmad, Jaleel. and A. H. Ashhar. *Unani: The Science of Graeco-Arabic Medicine*. New Delhi: Lustre Press Pvt. Ltd., 1998.

Barclay, Jane. "How Cold Was It?" Wiki, n.d. Accessed July 2017.

"Barefoot Doctor." *Wikipedia*. Wikimedia Foundation, March 6, 2020. Accessed March 2020. https:en.wikipedia.org/wiki/Barefoot_doctor.

Beebe, Signe. *Clinical Handbook of Chinese Veterinary Herbal Medicine*. New Mexico: Herbal Medicine Press, 2006.

Beinfield, Harriet and E. Korngold. *Between Heaven and Earth*. New York: Random House, 1991.

Bensky, Dan and R. Barolet. *Chinese Herbal Medicine Formulas & Strategies*. Seattle: Eastland Press, 1990.

Bensky, Dan and A. Gamble. *Chinese Herbal Medicine Materia Medica*. Seattle: Eastland Press, 1990.

Bisio, Tom. *A Tooth from the Tiger's Mouth*. New York: Simon and Schuster, 2004.

Bohm, David. *Wholeness and the Implicate Order*. New York: T.J. Routledge, 1995.

Capra, Fritjof. *The Systems View of Life*. New York: Cambridge University Press, 2018.

Capra, Fritjof. *The Tao of Physics*. Boston: Shambhala Publications, 1991.

Capra, Fritjof. *The Turning Point*. New York: Simon and Schuster, 1988.

Capra, Fritjof. *The Web of Life*. New York: Doubleday, 1996.

Chen, Ze-Lin and M. Chen. *A Comprehensive Guide to Chinese Herbal Medicine*. Long Beach: Oriental Healing Arts Institute, 1992

Sidel, Victor W, editor. A *Barefoot Doctor's Manual*. New York: Crown Publishers, 1985.

Chopra, Deepak. *Perfect Health*. New York: Random House, 2000.

Dalai Lama XIV. *The New Physics and Cosmology: Dialogues with the Dalai Lama*. New York: Oxford University Press, 2004.

Dossey, Larry. *Space, Time & Medicine*. Boston: Shambala Publications, 1989.

Feynman, Richard. *Six Easy Pieces: Essentials of Physics*. New York: Basic Books, 2011.

Frawley, David. *Ayurveda and the Mind*. 1997.

Frawley, David. *Ayurvedic Healing*. Twin Lakes: Lotus Press, 1989.

Frawley, David and V. Lad. *The Yoga of Herbs*, Twin Lakes: Lotus Press, 1988.

Gobbi, Marco 2001. "Pharmacopsychiatry." 45-8,34, no. Sup. 1 (July3, 2001). https://doi.org/10. 1055/s-002-1021.
Goswami, Amit. *The Self-Aware Universe.* New York: Putnam, 1995.
Goswami, Amit. *The Visionary Window, A Quantum Physicist's Guide to Enlightenment,* Wheaton, Illinois: Theosophical Publishing House, 2000.
Green, Barry. "Why is it that eating spicy, "hot" food causes the same physical reactions as does physical heat?" *Scientific American,* October 21, 1999.
Greger, Michael. *How Not to Die.* New York: Flatiron Books, 2015.
Grieve, Maude. 2014. *A Modern Herbal I.* New York: Dover Publications
Grieve, Maude. 2016. *A Modern Herbal II.* New York: Dover Publications
Griggs, Barbara. *Green Pharmacy.* New York: Viking Press, 1981.
Hammer, Leon. *Chinese Pulse Diagnosis, A Contemporary Approach.* Seattle: Eastland Press, 2001.
Heisenberg, Werner. *Physics and Philosophy, The Revolution in Modern Science.* New York: Harper & Row, 1962.
"Introduction to Quantum Mechanics." Wikipedia. Wikimedia Foundation. Accessed July 2017. https://en.wikipedia.org/wiki/Introduction_to_quantum _mechanics.
Johnson, Robert. "Ninety-Six Words for Love." *Awakin Weekly* September 15, 2014.
Kaptchuk, Ted. *The Web That Has No Weaver.* New York: Congdon & Weed, 1983.
Keown, Daniel. *The Spark in the Machine.* Philadelphia: Singing Dragon, 2014.
Kumar, Manjit. Quantum: Einstein, Bohr, and the great debate about the nature of reality. New York, N.Y., 2010.
Lad, Vasant. *A Complete Book of Ayurvedic Home Remedies.* Twin Lakes: Lotus Press, 1998.
Lad, Vasant. *Ayurvedic Perspectives on Selected Pathologies.* Twin Lakes: Lotus Press, 2012.
Lad, Vasant. *Ayurveda: The Science of Self Healing.* Wilmot: Lotus Light, 1985.
Lad, Vasant. *Textbook of Ayurveda: Volume 1.* Albuquerque: The Ayurvedic Press, 2002.
Lad, Vasant. *Textbook of Ayurveda Volume II: A complete Guide to Clinical Assessment.* Albuquerque: The Ayurvedic Press, 2006
Lad, Vasant. *Textbook of Ayurveda. Volume III.* Malaysia. 2012
Lakshmi, CM. editor. *Scientific Basis for Herbal Therapies.* Boca Raton: CRC Press, 2004.
Levy, Juliette. *The Complete Handbook for the Dog and Cat.* Great Britain: Mackays of Chatham, 1992.
Levy, Juliette. *Herbal Handbook for Farm and Stable.* Great Britain: Latimer Trend & Co., 1963.
Lu, H. C. *Chinese System of Food Cures.* New York: Sterling Publishing Co., 1986.
Maciocia, Giovanni. *The Foundations of Chinese Medicine.* Edinburgh: Churchill Livingstone, Robert Stevenson House, 2005
Maciocia, Giovanni. *Obstetrics and Gynecology in Chinese Medicine.* Edinburgh: Churchill Livingstone, Robert Stevenson House, 1998.
Maciocia, Giovanni. *The Practice of Chinese Medicine.* Edinburgh: Churchill Livingstone, Robert Stevenson House, 1997.
Manbiot, George. "How Wolves Change Rivers" YouTube. YouTube, November 15 2017. Accessed 2017. https://www.youtube.com./watch?v=oSBL7Gk_9QU.
Mastin Luke. "Physics of the Universe: Difficult Topics Made Understandable." Accessed July 2017. https://www.phsicsoftheuniverse.com/.

Metzner, Ralph. "The Causes of Disease: The Great Debate." Functional Medicine University—The Leader in Online Training in Functional Diagnostic Medicine July 17, 2014. https://functionalmedicineuniversity.com/public/937.cfm.

Naeser, Margaret. *Outline Guide to Chinese Herbal Patent Medicines in Pill Form.* Boston: Boston Chinese Medicine, 1992.

Ni, Maoshing. *The Tao of Nutrition.* Malibu: The Shrine of the Eternal Breath of Tao, 1989.

Niethammer, Carolyn. American Indian Food and Lore. New York: Collier, 1974.

Pole, Sebastian. *Ayurvedic Medicine.* Edinburgh: Churchill Livingstone, Robert Stevenson House, 2006

Remen, Rachel. "Helping, Fixing or Serving?" *Shambhala Sun,* September 1999.

Ridley, Matt. *Genome.* New York: Harper Collins, 2000.

Scheid, Volker, D. Bensky, A. Ellis, and R. Barolet. *Chinese Herbal Medicine Formulas and Strategies.* Seattle: Eastland Press, 2009.

Selbie, Joseph. *The Physics of God.* New Jersey: The Career Press, 2018.

Sheldrake, Rupert. *Science Set Free.* New York: Random House, 2012

Svoboda, Robert. *Ayurveda. Life, Health, & Longevity.* London: Penguin Group, 1992.

Svoboda, Robert. *Prakruti.* Twin Lakes: Lotus Press, 1998.

Svoboda, Robert. *Tao and Dharma. Chinese Medicine and Ayurveda.* Twin Lakes: Lotus Press, 1995.

"Theory of Relativity." *Wikipedia,* Wikimedia Foundation. Accessed April 2020. https://en.wikipedia.org/wiki/Theory_of_relativity.

Tierra, Michael. *Planetary Herbology.* Twin Lakes: Lotus Press, 1988.

Tierra, Michael. *The Way of Herbs.* New York: Simon & Schuster, 1983.

Tierra, Michael. *The Way of Chinese Herbs.* New York: Simon & Schuster, 1998.

Tompkins, Peter and C. Bird. *The Secret Life of Plants.* New York: Harper and Row, 1973.

Urantia Foundation. *The Urantia Book.* Chicago: Urantia Foundation, 1986.

Veith, Ilza. *The Yellow Emperor's Classic of Internal Medicine.* Los Angeles: University of California Press, 1972.

"What Is the Cloud-Definition: Microsoft Azure." Accessed March 2020. https://azure.microsoft.com/en-us/overview/what-is-the-cloud/.

World Health Organization Bulletin: China's village doctors take great strides. Volume 86: 2008. Number 12, December 2008, 909-988. Accessed March 2020. Who.int

Wu Bo-Ping and J Blalack. *Qin Bo-Wei's 56 Treatment Methods.* Seattle: Eastland Press, 2011

Yarema, Thomas, D. Rhoda and J. Brannigan. *Eat, Taste, Heal: An Ayurvedic Guidebook and Cookbook for Modern Living.* Kappa, Hawaii: Five Elements Press, 2006.

About the Author

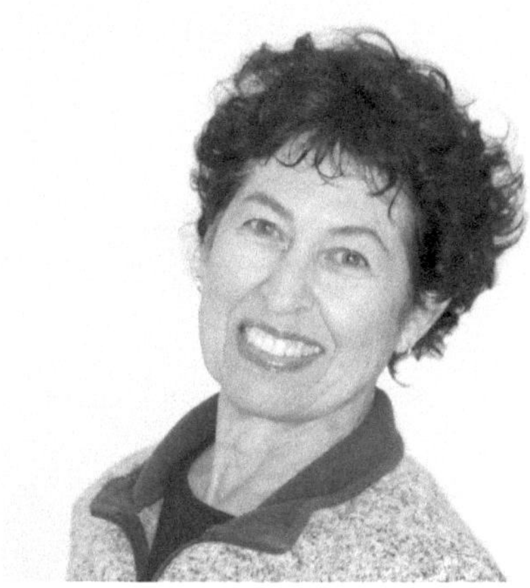

Judyth Shamosh, Ph.D., Systems Herbalist has been a continual student of herbal medicine since 1974. Clinical practitioner since 1994 and founder of Greenfingers Herbal Medicine Clinic, she practices Ayurvedic, Classical Chinese, and Western herbal medicine and teaches apprentices. She earned her undergraduate degree in the sciences and her Ph.D. in Natural Health. Dr. Judyth has studied with Rosemary Gladstar, Michael Tierra, Dr. Vasant Lad at the Ayurvedic Institute, and various teachers in Chinese medicine.

She has been a frequent lecturer of Ayurvedic and Classical Chinese herbal medicine at Phoenix Institute for Herbal Medicine & Acupuncture, on the governing council and current professional member of the American Herbalist's Guild, Vice Chairperson of the board at RainStar University College of Acupuncture and Oriental Medicine, on the adjunct faculty of the Southwest College of Naturopathic Medicine, the credentialing committee for the Arizona Center for Health and Medicine, Vice President of the Arizona Herb Association, assistant curator of the Phoenix Art Museum, geologist, archaeologist, festival coordinator, yoga instructor, and poet.